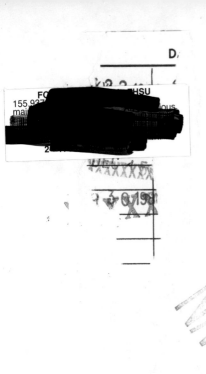

AN AMBITIOUS SORT OF GRIEF:

Woman, Reproduction, and Neo-Natal Loss

by

Marion Deutsche Cohen
Temple University

Mesquite   1983

Ide House

Published by
Ide House, Inc.
4631 Harvey Drive
Mesquite, Texas 75150-1609

Library of Congress Cataloging in Publication Data

Cohen, Marion Deutsche, 1943-
    An ambitious sort of grief.
     (Woman in history; ISSN 0195-9743 ; 72)
      1. Cohen, Marion Deutsche. 2. Mothers--Biography.
3. Children--Death. I. Title.
HQ759.C68 1983   155.9'37   83-8482
ISBN 0-86663-090-2 (lib. bdg.)
ISBN 0-86663-091-0 (pbk.)

Of the Ide House **Woman in history** series (ISSN 0195-9743), this is
Volume 72

October 25, 1977

The other day it occurred to me that I feel a bit phallic about my big belly. I mean, I'm conscious of it sticking out and I don't want to lose it. (This is *in addition* to the *pride* of being preg.) And I realize that I have a fear (well, a thought) that I'll be taken prisoner, along with a bunch of other people, and they'll put us all in this little teeny room, which *would* be large enough, if it weren't for my belly. Or they'll line us all up and have this big knife gradually descend, right in front of us—sort-of like *The Pit and the Pendulum*—placed so it *just* misses our noses, but not my belly. The idea is: Everyone *else* does okay, but not me. And not my baby!

I'm pretty sophisticated now, not like 'way back in high school. Not like the thirteen-year-old who dreamed she was married and she and her husband were in the kitchen and one of them said, 'Where are the kids?'' and the whole thing was so remote, soft-of, impossible, and shocking, almost. *Now* I really *have* been in the kitchen with my husband, and both of us *have* on occasion said, "Where are the kids?" and it is *not* inconsistent with "I exist" and all those other crazy adolescent feelings. Now I know how to live. Not I know how to act. NOW!

But sometimes things still confuse me. Sometimes I'm definitely out of it. Like the other day, we were all sitting on the park bench—me, Jeff, Barbara, and Anita (our two new-neighborhood friends). And I had my hand on my stomach—I always have my hand on my stomach when I'm preg , even before I'm sure I'm preg. I walk around with my hand on my belly. So now I had my hand on my belly and Barbara asked, "Is the baby active today?"

And once again I was confused. Once again I was out of it. Am I supposed to have my hand on my stomach only when the baby's moving? And am I supposed to be doing it only to sort-of hold my stomach together?

I was lost in these thoughts for a few seconds and then, just as the time was almost up for answering, I said, "Oh no, not at all. *I'm* active today."

If all mothers had natural birth, totally breast-fed, didn't wean 'til three years if at all, left their older kids in day care, or with baby-sitters, or (better yet) without baby-sitters, wrote poems about pushing, and gave Politics of Motherhood workshops at women's centers and bookstores—if all mothers did these things—then I suppose maybe I wouldn't enjoy motherhood as much.

Recurring dreams:

1.   We're having a family get-together and my father is there, usually sitting on the chair opposite me and half-smiling. "This is a dream," I tell him, "because you're dead." He remains half-smiling. I begin to mold his face.

2.   I have a baby and the labor and delivery are so short and easy that I sleep through it. When I wake up I feel cheated and unsure that the baby lying at the foot of the bed is mine. I keep leaving it places and forgetting to feed it. When I remember, I feel sad. The feeling is *not* only of guilt.

3.   I have a baby which is beautiful but very big, about the size of a two-year-old.

4.   I have two babies in rapid succession (say, less than a year apart).

5.   I tell my mother off. It's entirely realistic.

6.   I have the same childlike lonely monogamous feelings but am unattached.

October 27, 1977

Today Elle said two things that make me proud of her, and of me: (1) She said "All the black kids in my class like me. 'Cause I say things like '*I* think its okay to have different colored people in the world'." (2) Although she and her friends do oogle over Shaun Cassidy and his "Do Run Run" song (as I've said before, she *will* have to try it out), there's this one part she was singing—something like "She makes me feel so fine"—after which she said, ' See? That's okay, right, Ma? That's not sexist. A woman singing about another woman. 'She makes me feel so fine.' So the song is for lesbians, too, right?"

Last night I had a good cry. I haven't had one of those for a long time. It must have been largely a pregnancy-hormonal mood because I don't feel at all like crying this morning. But: it does really seem that no one ever *remembers* me. I have to keep *reminding* them.

It started with the baby-shower business. This is my third baby and I still haven't gotten a baby shower. I have a few—certainly enough—*good* friends but I don't have a circle of friends—ya know, a bunch of people all of whom are friendly with each other. That seems to make the difference. F— did promise me—four years ago when I discussed it with her just after having Arin—that she'd give me a shower with my next baby. And I did remind her of it, and I keep reminding Jeff to call her up and remind her and plan it with her. (No one ever remembers me, they all have to be reminded.) But Jeff is sick and F— is busy (finally writing her PhD thesis). R— is due this week herself, and J— and W— are probably too political. Jeff's family gives bridal, not baby showers, and my mother doesn't approve of any of it.

Elle caught my mood a few weeks ago, and kept whispering to Jeff about it, but I'm sure she's also forgotten it by now. Jeff says he'll try to get F— to do it, or cover for him so *he* can do it, but I don't know. He keeps asking *me* questions. How can F— do it when she lives out of town? If F— won't do it, who else will? It seems I'm the smartest one in the world when it comes to making baby showers. (Just as, when I'm sick, the family does eat, but not quite as well.)

Question: What does God do when she or he has a hankering to be given a surprise party?

Yes, it has to be a surprise. Like Robin's. Now, *she* was really surprised. She didn't even suspect. Her husband just up and took her out for shopping and lunch and when she returned, there we all were. She didn't have to think about it, or wonder about it, or remind people about herself. They simply remembered. It just happened.

16 years ago, my bridal shower was *al*most a surprise. But my father ruined it. He and I were alone in the house while my mother and Rozzy were out on some pretense, and I was waiting for Jeff to pick me up and supposedly take me out to dinner. And the 'phone rang downstairs and my father answer-

ed it while I was getting dressed and I guess the person must have asked for my mother or Rozzy because I heard him say, in his typical big booming voice, "*I* don't know, she's at *some shower* or something."

"*Some* shower." He also doesn't approve of these things. "Some shower." I still don't know whether or not he did it purposedly. He's dead now, but I would never have known, anyway. "Some shower." My only chance to be surprised. I feel cheated.

And "the girls at the office" can't make me a shower because there *are* no "girls at the office." Yes, this is another unemployment-year for me. Temple and Drexel didn't remember me, either. (And I called them both twice, to remind them.) I was hoping it would be different this time. I was hoping to be able to tell my roommate, "Well, yes, I'm teaching a course at Temple," or, "I'll be going back to work in two or three weeks."

The poetry places didn't remember me either. I gave so many readings last year and none of them called me back. W— and I are working our heads off with this anthology, and none of the influential women who are in it have done any of *us* a damn bit of good. K.B. said she was gonna invite me to read at P.B., and R.L. said she was gonna call me about reading at McG's, but I don't know. . . I just bet they don't call. It has to *happen*; don't you understand. It has to *happen*, and it just never does. I have to keep *making* it happen. I have to keep *reminding* them.

It's as though I'm gonna have this baby and no one cares. It's like, as I've said before, it's like a mother and her baby are alone in the world. Six hours after the birth, they want me to start bathing. Both me and the baby. I don't *want* to wash off the meconium. I'm still giving birth and they don't understand that. I'm not a regular mother yet; it's like I'm still pregnant. The baby's skin is still tingling from contact with my insides, and my perineum. It's like the afterglow of an orgasm. And it lasts for months.

I've done so many things in my life; why can't any of it pay off? Oh, I *know* why—because I don't have a circle of friends, because I'm different, because I'm radical, because the majority is always wrong. I *know* why, but that doesn't make it any easier. Why can't even one person appreciate me enough

to make me a baby shower? Even one. I'm not asking for the
majority. Just one.

In my usual "cute" way, I've made a complete list for Jeff
and F— & Co. Who I wanted invited, 'phone numbers and ad-
dresses, even what I want for presents, and what I *don't* want,
plus a reminder to "don't tell the kids until the last minute; I
want it to be a surprise." But God can't get surprises—can it?

P.S. It's not that I en*joy* pitying myself. It's that I have learned
to enjoy it. I've learned to get something out of it. I'd much
rather not have to; I'd much rather just plain-ol' be surprised,
like Robin.

Put another way, as in poems I've written. "I wish I were
masochistic" or "Sure, women are masochistic; we've got no
choice."

October 31, 1977

Once more a publisher has expressed an interest in my
"Motherhood" book. Will I be disappointed again? Is this a
trick or treat?! (Note date.)

The 8th month—savoring the luxury of resting things on
top of my belly (hands, packages, the waistlines of Mexican
tops).

Just because it would be *nice* if there were a God, doesn't
mean there is a God.

And who says it would be nice if there were a God?

Deep down inside people must know that, besides harbor-
ing "faith" in good, they must also harbor "faith" in bad. Say-
ings like "tempting Providence" and superstitions like about
walking under a ladder or stepping on a crack plus all the fears
that we readily admit to at night attest to that. Deep down inside people know that, even if there is a God, it might not be all
good.

When people say they believe in God, what they're really
saying is "Hey, let's *pretend* there's a God."

Nancy says she believes in God again because she now realizes, through psychoanalysis, that the reason she started rejecting God in the first place was that she was rejecting the father image. Possibly true, but that doesn't mean there *is* a God. And what about the reason she started *believing* in God in the first place?

I've forgotten again—I always do—the ecstasy I'm going to feel *right after* having the baby. Reading the two birth diaries won't help; I won't know again until it happens. Once again I'll be surprised.

Elle is as excited as though she were an adult, and not at all jealous. She puts her arms around my stomach, loving me and the baby together. "We *know* it's cute," I say. "We don't know what it looks like, but we *know* it's cute."

Fantasy: As firemen proceed to rescue two young children from a burning house, the mother, from the crowd and from the depths of her subconscious, screams, "Get the baby first! Get the baby first!"

Why do people persist in thinking that the way to calm a crying baby is to give it the ol' pep talk—ya know, bounce it around, shake a rattle, pinch its cheek? It doesn't surprise me to see adults treat each *other* that way, but I still can't get over it when they do it with babies, too.

I love to eat out when I'm preg. I don't know; it just seems to me that . . . I don't know. . . that the occasion is more *festive* somehow.

Even though this time I'm more excited about the actual baby than any of the other times, I'm going to miss this one after it's born, too.

This time I'm not gonna hafta lie awake after delivery and having this nagging thought return to me the morning after that I'm not Doing Anything Right Now. This time I've just edited a local women's poetry anthology and my Math Anxiety Workshop is written up in the Temple catalog for February and, about a month before my due date, I went into New York to meet with the publisher of my first book, plus just about two weeks ago, I got a letter from the possible (*very* possible, it would seem) publisher of my second book. My Politics of Motherhood book! Now, *that* would *really* make my year. Plus I'm pretty much rid of the Doing Things hang-up, anyway.

PLUS I got my baby shower!

It was two days ago. One of the big things in my life. Jeff called up W— (who co-edited the women's anthology with me) and asked her to make it for me. She was happy to, and when they got to calling up F— and inviting *her*, F— told Jeff, "Hey, from now, I'm taking over."

So my friends didn't exactly do it on their own—a lot of reminding had to be done—but they sure did get into the spirit once they did do it. And now, of course, F— and W— are great friends (So I have, if not a *circle* of friends, at least two points, which make a *line*!)

It certainly put me on a good friend-ego trip and I certainly felt popular and loved. And I realized that I do, in a sense, have a circle of friends. I mean, so many of them are Philadelphia poets, and they do all know each other (most of them are in the anthology). Another thing that made me feel good: my mother took me aside and exclaimed, in wonder, "Your friends *love* you. They really *love* you."

I even had a small dyke contingent! B.A., G—, her lover B——although my really good dyke friend J— didn't arrive until everyone else left. But there they all were, in the midst of my baby shower and all Jeff's relatives. I felt very proud indeed—so whole, so non-heterosexist. Like I did that time walking into Giovanni's Room (the gay/feminist book store) with Arin plus a big belly plus my anthology to consign. It's just so neat. I think this pregnancy has done a lot for my heterosexual-guilt, or whatever other hang-up I might have concerning being a married radical feminist. I mean, the dykes know I'm preg and they approve. Actually, they seem to more than approve. I just think the whole thing's fun. Maybe I shouldn't but I do.

Anyway, the shower turned out really nice. Elle made pictures and hung them up over the presents. The pictures had messages on them, messages on the order of "Cry baby. Don't have a cry baby," and "I like babies but don't have a cry baby." Typical of Elle. And her friend Jill wrote, "I hope you have a girl." And Arin drew a picture which is really good;

Wemara described it as being like Miro.

Elle and I were both really excited about the presents and at first I let all the kids help me open them. But then they started fighting over the packages and opening them all at the same time in general not enjoying themselves as much as initially. Nor was it the way *I* wanted things, either. So I asked if someone would please take the kids away; and someone did. It worked out fine. The Politics of Motherhood came in very handy.

And the presents were great. Not all Carter's little printed undershirts, and nothing from Born Yesterday, but no junk, either. Let's see—a blanket with a cat pillow, another blanket, a yellow "bunny suit", as I call them, newborn Pampers, Carter's printed carriage sheets, one crib sheet, two stretch suits, one "Super-Baby" undershirt, one "Bebe" undershirt, (both with pants), a sweater and hat set, two printed undershirts, two plain, a book of Shakespeare rewritten for kids (Charles and Mary Lamb), three books for *me* (although I actually would have preferred more things for the baby), and a book of poetry *from* W——— , *by* W———, and *for* Jeff, me, and baby. There must be more, but I can't remember.

Anyway, I got my shower.

"One thing I'm *not* gonna do," I tell Elle and Arin, "is make like those nervous guilt-ridden mothers who, for fear their kids might get jealous or something, call the baby '*our* baby'. I mean, it *is* partially your baby, but it was Daddy and I who decided to have it. And I know you want it, too, but we'd have it even if you didn't. And mainly, *I'm* the one whose stomach it's in and I'm the one who's gonna push it out. *Our* baby, my foot! If I lived in a commune, I'd probably write a 'run-on' poem which began 'Whaddaya mean, the collective baby?!' "

In the B— waiting room: How could that mother, over there in the corner nursing her four-week old, *not* say things like, "You *like* t'eat? You *like* your food? Is it good? You're so yummy. You're absolutely delicious. You're just as *nice* as can be." How can she avoid a lingo; how can she talk to her friend in a perfectly normal tone. How can she be so damn calm?

December 2, 1977

I just this minute found out: the baby has dropped. I really can't believe it; twice I said to the midwife, "So the baby's actually dropped?" See, both my previous babies dropped an hour or so before being born. As I say, "they didn't drop until they dropped *out*." So I really can't believe it.

Neither of us *like* the idea of a baby dropping, actually. We don't like the idea of its head being held in one position for so long, being imprisoned like that. *My* head gets sort-of dizzy at night if I don't move it enough.

It seems this baby is a horse (pony?) of a different color. I had really bad morning sickness—was in bed for three months—had a lot of faint-ness, had an ear-ache, a sinus infection, and now I have a cold which won't go away, a vaginal infection, and all my pelvic and upper leg joints are stiff. I'm not calling it a "difficult pregnancy", it's just that plenty of things have been annoying. This is also the first "vitamin baby"; I lapse a lot, but in general I'm taking multiple vitamin and minerals, B complex, kelp, E, wheat germ, dolomite, and, of course, C. This just might be a super-baby! And also. this time the midwife said it seems like "nice-sized babies"—seven and three-quarter pounds, she estimates. Elle was five pounds four teen ounces and Arin was six pounds seven ounces. *Also*, in my opinion, "nice-sized babies"—but it *would* be fun to hit seven pounds. I'm not especially big; most people say I certainly don't look like I'm due next week. But I did gain two and a half pounds this week.

Yes, this baby just might be a horse of a different color.

Two ways in which I hope it *isn't* a horse of a different color: (1) I hope there isn't anything wrong with it. (2) I hope I don't have a long labor, or a complicated delivery.

Elle informs friends of ours, "Hey, today the baby *fell*"!

December 16, 1977

I thought this baby would come on time but I guess not. It was due Dec. 11, and we *are* sure of the conception day. I thought at least it wouldn't come any later than Arin, who was 4 days late, but I guess it has.

Yes, there has been some action. Braxton-Hicks all week, starting a week ago. Sometimes they'll even come 10 minutes apart for the space of an hour or two, but they don't fool me! I know they're only bluffing.

With Arin, they actually hurt, but these don't. I don't know whether it's because I'm taking mega-doses of calcium and vitamin C, or whether it's just because "every pregnancy is different".

This is the first time I've ever been conscious of the due date, and of waiting. I'm finding it sort-of fun! I'm not at all uncomfortable but I am a bit impatient. Probably because *Elle* is so excited. Every day, she tells me, on her way home from school she sings a little song which goes, "Make the baby be born, make the baby be born, and make it be a girl!" Some mornings she greets me with "Did you have any contractions last night?" As I said, this is the first time I find myself waiting, and it's fun! I find myself joking about it and all.

I also feel—yep, I admit it—a bit nervous. *Also* for the first time. Just a bit. I'm nervous about how long it'll take, and I'm nervous about the episiotomy, of all things, and I'm nervous that I won't feel the same ecstasy I felt after the other births. I'm even nervous that there'll be something wrong with the baby. How blase can ya get?!

Also for the first time, I'm excited about the baby itself, *i.e.*, I *believe* in the baby itself. I find myself staring fixedly at all the "coming-home" babies and "four-weeks-appointment" babies at B—, and I find myself dreaming up every excuse I can to go into the "baby's room"—the little linen room in our house, where we keep the baby's clothes. But lately, when I come home with a new bundle from the thrift shop, Elle's not that thrilled. It's the baby she wants. "I like babies better than baby clothes," she says. "Don't you, mommy?"

I answer, "Sometimes I wonder!"

Whenever the 'phone rings I find myself half-expecting it

to be someone informing us that Marion had her baby!

One night I had these Braxton-Hicks regular and strong (but not hurting) for about two hours. Before they ceased and I dropped off to sleep, I had all kinds of neat thoughts and I was gonna get up and write them down (but was too lazy). "In the wee hours of labor," I was gonna write, "I find myself thinking about Sartre's novel *Nausea*. Of all things! Thinking about existence when you're in labor! It exists, the baby exists, it all exists. And I'm so glad it does! Solipsism is quite another thing—wish I'd never heard of it! I think of a 'tidbit' I once wrote; it goes, 'Who is the solipsist, the mother or the child?' I also think of another poem of mine which I haven't written down yet, called 'Solipsist in Labor'. This poem I apologize for, because (1) I'm not a solipsist, but I have a solipsist streak, as possibly everyone has, (2) the poem doesn't represent my most intense feelings, and (3) it's unfair to the baby. The poem goes—well, it's something like this:

> *Did I push out the* other *things, too?*
> *Did it take long?*
> *The chairs, the table—how long ago was it?*
> *Do I love them, too, and have I forgotten?*

or something like that."

I was gonna write all that down, and probably more, but I was too lazy. Maybe if I *had* gotten up, the baby would have been born.

December 19, 1977

Even the Braxton-Hicks have stopped. Yup, even they've given up! What they were doing before is engaging the baby's head, and now that that's done, apparently they feel they've done enough. People say, "Maybe it's not *in* there," but I *feel* it in there, alive and kicking. Each day I go to more thrift shops and buy more clothes for it, and in the past few days I've made three appliqued quilts for it, but apparently none of this has tempted it. Even the weather warming up hasn't helped. Jeff says it likes all the vitamins and iron and raita and seven-grain bread I'm feeding it, and apparently it doesn't know about dp-dp-dp (my lingo for nursing). The grandparents gave up and came in to see us the day before yesterday, bearing Chanukah presents for Elle and Arin, a nightgown with buttons down the front for me, Arin's old bassinette, a pot roast, cold cuts, and other assorted goodies. We had fantasized about that being the day but it wasn't.

This delay is a nice interlude for me; I feel great physically, I make no plans, I often nap in the afternoon, I walk, I relax, I absorb the fact of my pregnancy. I *should* clean the house but I don't feel like it. I also should make the cushions for the living room chair, but I don't feel like that either. I don't even particularly feel like writing. I feel very pleasure-oriented—lazy, in a sense—but only in a sense. I feel like a lady-in-waiting. For a while there, when I had the Braxton-Hicks, I felt like I was living from one hour to the next, now I only feel I'm living from one *day* to the next. Our meals are unplanned, especially since my afternoon naps are usually *late* afternoon naps. Sometimes Jeff and Elle will make a salad—consisting of coarsely cut-up vegetables (that's putting it kindly!) and tuna fish or sour cream and toast. Sometimes we send the kids out to Jack Kramer's Deli around the corner while we have our raita and curried vegetables.

Ya know, I never knew that parents thought their kids were *cute*. I mean, before Elle was born, I always assumed parents merely *loved* their kids, but were too *used* to them to find them cute. Know what I mean? And I guess I might have also believed that loving and thinking-cute were contradictory, and that, in my present jargon, cuteness was oppressive.

But the more I love Elle and Arin, the cuter I think they are. And I find nursing babies, and newborn babies, and *un*born babies, the cutest of all. So I can't bring myself to say cuteness is oppressive—any more, I guess, than I can believe that female-ness or child-ness is oppressive. It's the world's *image* of these things—cute, female, and child—that becomes oppressive.

I have certain feelings about the way men feel about preg-nant women. Especially swinging single men. I mean, to *them* I'm probably completely non-sexual—which is, to them, non-existent. I don't know. . . I can't explain it, exactly. Unim-portant, that's the word. To them I'm probably unimportant. Like, they probably know, in their conscious minds, that I'm beautiful, but I'm not the kind of beautiful *they*'re interested in. Like, they're in a different world. I don't know. . . it's vague.
Of course, I also realize that there are men who get turned on by pregnant women. F—— once said her husband thinks pregnant women are sexy. I wonder. He might mean sensual. I don't know. . . This whole sexy or sensual business just doesn't send me. I guess I don't want to be either sexy *or* sens-ual. To me, both words have too many sexist associations. I like old-fashioned flannel nightgowns and ethnic clothing and meconium-stained hospital-maternity-ward gowns.

I think it would be neat to write a poem called "Ode to a Labor Contraction" and read it at my next reading. But I don't have any ideas as to what the poem would say that was new, or whether or not it would be political in any way, or what, in fact, to say at all.

December 20, 1977

A few Braxton-Hicks today, but they're not particularly strong. Am I creating them? A true "Solipsist in Labor"!

I feel a little as though I'm being stood up by a friend on a luncheon date.

December 21, 1977

I also feel a little like I did when I was a teen-ager and couldn't get dates. So many times, it seemed, I almost had a date, but then the guy never called. So I would get all nervous at first and then, after a week or so, I would relax and say to myself, bitterly, "There's no reason to be nervous. You're not going to have a date."

Now I say to myself, "There's no reason to be nervous. You're not going to have a baby."

And also, listen to what *else* happened that's *also* like my not being able to get dates as a teen-ager. Remember my entry of Oct. 31? Well, it was a trick.

Another trick. Once again, God fooled me. Made it seem like something good was gonna happen and then made it not happen. It really did seem they were gonna publish that motherhood book, but today I got the letter saying no. They want me to not be coming from the perspective of white middle-class, plus they don't like the first person, plus they think it's too moralistic sounding. At least that's what they say. The point is: *Another* no. I had tried not to get all excited about it but I guess God can read thoughts. And s/he did it again. The probability was over 50% but s/he dished me out another no. And right around baby-time, too. Like a child, I ask, "How can s/he be so cruel?" Crazy, of course. S/he's been crueler than that, to other people. I mean, imagine being in a concentration camp for four years and then finally getting out and finding your entire family dead. There's no end to how cruel God can be. But does that mean that, no matter how cruel s/he is to *me*, I haven't the right to complain?

I *won't* cheer myself up by looking at the bassinette. Then God'll make something go wrong with the baby.

The thing I can't bear is that the *probability* was that they would accept. And I keep comparing the way I feel with the way I *would* feel if that letter *had* been an acceptance.

It's a letdown. It's a tragedy. A tragedy. NO less than if someone had died.

December 26, 1977

I was wrong, of course (referring to the above). Some*one* dying is worse than some*thing* dying. Oh horror! O! horror! It is a nightmare worse.

Because you're not going to *believe this* one. I'll be as brief as possible, then fill in the details later: on the morning of December 22, the day after the rejection letter, Jeff and I mailed off my answer to S.E. Press, went to the bank, picked up the crib mattress plus some upholstery zippers, then settled down to lunch in a cozy expensive one-shot deal kind of place. Well, just after we ordered, I felt my water break. This time, I decided, I'd first check in the ladies' room and then come back and surprise Jeff. I had it all planned. But when I checked in the ladies' room, what I saw was not water but this thick greenish stuff, which I figured was probably meconium, because there'd been meconium with the other two births. There were no contractions, no pain, and in happy anticipation I 'phoned B—. Just for completeness' sake, but not because I believed it was important, I told them about the meconium, also that I was almost two weeks late. I wasn't worried, and B— didn't seem worried, but of course, since the water had broken, they said I could come in. At first I wanted to cancel our order but then Jeff said, "Remember what Adelle Davis says," and I recalled the fragment from her chapter "For an easier delivery". . . .*a hearty snack of bread, milk, fruit, and cheese at the onset of labor...* We had ordered French onion soup, salads, and a cheese omlet. "I may be in labor," I told the waiter, "so could we cancel the entree and just keep the appetizers?" He was one of those "ti-ti" (as we say) waiters and with absolutely no facial expression he answered "surely" and we laughed. We quickly ate the food, which wasn't all that great, then picked up Arin at Durham, met Elle back home, arranged for my friend Elaine to pick up the kids around 5:00 or 6:00 and have them sleep over, called B— again (Jeff wasn't sure we should come in because I was having virtually no contractions) and proceeded on our way. Elle sent me off with a hug on the belly, Arin with an indifferent shrug.

It was probably the best early labor I have ever had. In the car, the contractions quickly regularized to every three minutes, short and completely painless. (With Arin, these early ones were painful.) I'd been drinking 1½ quarts of milk a day plus taking vitamin E, also from that Adelle Davis chapter, so I had no pain and very little apprehension. We passed a new thrift shop on the way, and I *was* in the mood for going inside, but we figured we'd better hurry up because of the meconium. But, as I said, I wasn't really worried because Elle had swallowed meconium, had had to be resuscitated, and in 5 or 10 minutes was just fine. We realized that we had forgotten to take the vitamin C and E with us, so we bought some on the way. I remember I stayed inside the car while Jeff went into the drugstore because, . . . I don't know. . . somehow I *did* feel nervous, and, while he was inside, I took out the stethoscope and checked the heartbeat (the baby's). It was there, and I felt relieved, but it seemed to me it was slow, but I figured I wasn't the doctor and probably just wasn't hearing it right, or maybe it was supposed to be slow. Anyway, I remember that I didn't tell Jeff about this little incident, and I normally tell him everything. I think a part of me wanted my doubts not to be there.

Anyway, almost as soon as we arrived at B—, they put me on the fetal heart monitor. I didn't realize at the time, but they weren't particularly pleased with what they found. The beat was extremely variable, ranging from 79 to 200 something. I was 2 centimeters, half-effaced, and contracting often but not strongly. They connected me to an internal monitor, kept giving me oxygen, and told me if I didn't proceed fast enough they'd give me pitocin. They knew about my history of short labors, so they didn't rush things. It was about 4:00 when we had arrived. The contractions were perfectly painless until, say, about 5:30. That was when Jeff called Elle to tell her to go over to Elaine's. The 'phone was right in the room. I remember him saying, "No, not yet, but we're making progress. . . Three, so far. . . No, she has to get to ten. . . No, she can't come to the 'phone. She's not allowed to. . . " Of course, I was. I was just afraid to talk to her during a contraction. Oh yes, I had decided to start my "walking method"—of course, I could only pace a small area, being attached to the monitor—and that was keeping the heart rate higher (but not high enough) and also making the contractions stronger. In general, they were irregular in strength, and some involved more pressure than others. They were 1½ minutes apart and lasted 30-40 seconds, even shorter than in my previous two labors. Each strong one, however, was a noticeable mite stronger than the previous strong one; it seemed as though each one dilated me, say, half a centimeter. By 6:00 I was 5½ centimeters and she stretched me to 6, saying, "I don't usually believe in doing this, but in this case I do." I don't know the time lapse, but it didn't seem long before I started in with the "I hafta go to the bathroom" bit. "Oh, that would be great if it was the baby," said Dr. M———. "I don't think it's the baby," I said. "I know the difference." But after the next contraction I told her, "It's the baby." But I added, "I don't have the urge to push, though." Then suddenly someone was saying, "Have her lie on her side," and then I was on my side and breathing oxygen again and I heard the monitor dropping, dropping, and I panicked but did as I was told—breathed the oxygen slowly and deeply, instead of doing the transitional breathing I should have been doing and letting Elle hold my leg up while Dr. M— stretched me from 9½ to 10 centimeters, and somehow at the same time, screaming—or rather, moaning at the intensity of a scream. "Open your eyes," E — kept saying; and then, "Listen, we're taking you into the D.R."

I'd never heard the term "D.R." before, but you can be sure I knew what it meant. "Great," I said—then "Oh baby! baby!" "Sorry I'm being such a bad patient," I added. "Oh, now listen," responded Dr. M———, "One thing I can't stand is apologies." "I usually don't apologize," I answered, "but somehow this time I'm finding that screaming is more helpful than breathing!"

I was all set for happiness. I forgot about the meconium. I forgot about the monitor. I thought only of the baby about to be born. "If it doesn't hurt to push—*push*," urged Dr. M———; so, although I had no urge, I pushed. It all happened so fast. As I said, there was no urge to push. And pushing brought no relief, no pleasure, like the other times. Nor could I feel the progress I was making. I pushed in between contractions, too; I just kept pushing. I felt as though nothing was happening, but Dr. M——— kept saying, "Good." I even had to ask, "Is the head out?"

"Yes, the head's out," she told me; but I still wasn't satisfied. "Better remind me not to push," I gasped and started blowing like mad, because, although with Arin I had no urge to push after his head came out, this time I felt as though I were still in transition. *My* body knew: that baby hadda come out!

But Dr. M—— said something like, "Whaddaya mean, tell you not to push. Go ahead and push," and, for a second there, I actually was blowing and pushing at the same time.

The whole birth couldn't have taken more than a minute. It felt more like 5 seconds. And, once it was over, there I was, in ectasy, shouting out again, "Baby! Oh, baby! baby!"

As with Elle, at first I didn't notice that the baby wasn't crying. And I certainly didn't notice that she was blue. And I *certainly* didn't notice that her heart-rate, pulse, everything was a total of zero, but that she had somehow kicked her little baby leg.

It took me, say, five seconds to realize that they had put her on the table, instead of on my stomach, and were working feverishly on her. "Just like Elle," I said. I really believed that. But another part of me kept guard. "Oh, please let her be all right. Please let the little girl be all right." Jeff and I just stayed there the whole time and held hands, and, to tell the truth, kind-of enjoyed the whole delivery room atmosphere despite the circumstances.

She had been born at 7:07. It was around 11:00 when they transferred her to Jefferson Hospital. Her heart rate they had gotten up—it was now plenty high and steady. Sometimes she breathed on her own; usually she didn't. They told us they didn't know whether she would live. On the other hand, Dr. M—— came over to us and said, "Personally, I think she's going to be fine. I could be wrong, though."

The problem was with her lateness. Funny, how I had had a slight apprehension about it—just oh, so slight, though. But it was the first time during a pregnancy that I felt that way, even a little. She was late, and she matured early. The pediatrician called her "old"; he said she looked about three weeks old. The main problem was that the umbilical cord had shriveled and it was hard for her to get oxygen; hence, the stress—hence, the meconium. Other complications had arisen from that; her bladder, her kidneys, perhaps also her brain. "She's a real fighter," they commented as they worked on her. "And she's cute, too. Look at her little pointy chin." "Like Elle," I said.

I cried a little after they transferred her to Jefferson, and I collected my wits, realizing she might not live through the night—but I still spent that night in my typical post-partum happiness. You know, thinking about the pushing and the little head and then the little body—and *baby*! baby!

Around 2:00 I rang for a sleeping pill, realizing I would need my strength for the next day—when I would be discharged from B— and visiting Kerin at Jefferson. So I slept well 'til about 7:00 or so—when I woke up nervous. When someone came in, it was to tell me that Kerin was alive but not well, and that I should call the hospital soon and see how she was doing. So I just turned over and began sobbing, and Mrs. F—, one of the midwives, came in and said, "I'm so sorry, dear," and asked if there was anything she could do. "Yes," I answered, "dial my husband's number". I dictated it, and she got Jeff for me. "Please get over here as soon as you can," I sobbed into the 'phone. "They say the baby's not doing too well and we should call the hospital and . . . I just can't handle it." So he came over and I had breakfast and got dressed and we talked to my roommate and sort-of pretended everything was really all right.

And so I got to wear my going-home dress, which I'd made from Guatemalaen fabric; that was all I unpacked from my suitcase. And I left B— sans baby—you know, the whole bit—and we went to Jefferson to visit Kerin.

I thought she looked great, but they told us there wasn't much hope. "She's a very sick baby," they said. I cried several times.

Like any new mother, I was just a little shy at this first visit. I found I could pet her easily but not talk to her—not as much as I wanted to. I certainly didn't find the same joy as I did on the second visit—later that night.

Neither of us could tear ourselves away from her. We talked to her, played with her; I felt at peace just touching her arms and looking at her. Elle had a message for her; it was either "Get better, little sister," or, "Come home. little sister." I forget which; I gave Kerin both messages.

Kerin stretched her baby arms when we touched her, and half-opened her baby eyes (which were blue). Just before we left, we noticed that she also moved in response to our voices—both of ours. I'm sure it wasn't our imagination. Somewhere, somehow, she recognized us from the nine-plus months.

I wished we had stayed longer. It was 2:30 a.m., and I had just delivered the previous night—and Jeff was sick. Still we wish we had stayed longer. "We'll see you tomorrow," I told her. "I'll bring you a present." I had noticed that some of the other babies had toys in their little incubators in the intensive care unit, and I had in mind the little orange baby kangeroo I had brought. (It went inside its mother kangeroo, but the mother was too big for the incubator.) "Good-bye, little sweetie," I told her. "I'll see you tomorrow; I can't guarantee the morning; we're gonna be pretty tired. But we'll come see you just as soon as we can, sweetheart. Your's sooo sweet." Plenty of tears, but I was so happy. I was beginning to get into the spirit of having this baby in the intensive care unit to visit.

I had a good sleep that night (but Jeff later told me he cried in the bathroom before *he* went to sleep). In the morning (I had no idea what time) I kept hearing the 'phone ring and going rigid and listening and hearing nothing and being afraid it was the hospital calling to tell us the worst and burrowing deeper under the covers and falling back to sleep—and in general being afraid to go downstairs for fear of what they would tell me. So by the time I *did* go downstairs (and I did so only because I could hear everyone talking normally) it was 2:15 p.m.; I hadn't realized it was so late and I was anxious to go see Kerin. But not anxious enough, I feel. I didn't go rush right out; I sat down to relax and be served breakfast.

"Hilda called the hospital," my mother told me in that way of hers that dissolves *all* question as to whether everything is gonna be fine. "Hilda called the hospital, and they say her condition is stable." Oh, whew! I thought. "Also," she continued, "Faygie called Solly (my uncle who's a doctor), and he says he's not too worried. Of course, he won't give a definite opinion without seeing the patient, but he says once these babies get over the first few days they're usually perfectly fine." Etc., etc..

I was made to feel almost *casual* about the whole thing. I *wanted* to feel almost casual about the whole thing. So I relaxed and ate breakfast; then, around 3:00, I prepared to go to the hospital with Jeff.

Jeff decided to call them first. They told him that she was stable (*i.e.* her heartbeat), but that her urine was black and her kidneys were bad, that she'd been nice and pink for about two hours that morning, and had had no "seizures". (To Jeff and me, that meant no arm and leg movements and we considered that bad news.) As usual, they were far from optimistic, and after Jeff hung up he told us, "He had to go 'cause one of the emergency buzzers went off; he said he'd call me back." "Not necessarily *Kerin's* buzzer," he added; "just some buzzer."

"Oh, I know," I said, almost laughing. "Those buzzers are *constantly* going off, and its always something wrong with the machine or something." Although I had my coat on, I went upstairs to have my first B.M. since delivery. Sitting on the toilet, and feeling pretty good, I heard the 'phone ring. I froze only a little this time. And then—and then. . . .

Oh God! this is going to be hard to write! But I have written things that were hard to write before.

And then—I heard a gasp and some sobs and my mother crying out—Oh God!—"The baby's gone!"

I cry as I write this, but that's nothing new. I cry all the time; I'm miserable; my milk comes in right now; I am so sad and disappointed; Jeff is the same—and we are all having trouble living. At the same time I must have turned white but I remembered to walk slowly down the stairs and hold on to the bannister. I found a bunch of waiting arms for me in the kitchen and chose Jeff's. Once there, I emitted several unearthly sounds, resembling the sounds I made during delivery only in their unearthliness. And then we were all just *there*, Jeff's mother and mine pacing separately, in tears, Jeff and I clinging to each other. I felt sorry for my mother pacing alone so I grabbed her hand for a second but eventually everyone left Jeff and me in the room. And then, for the very first time, I saw Jeff cry.

He wanted a funeral, and I wanted to be with him, so there was a short simple ceremony the next morning. She was named Janey Kerin Suzanne, the Janey after my father Jack, and also after the "Janey dolls" of my early childhood. She was buried in a crypt which my parents had purchased ages ago—but which they had changed their minds about, deciding to leave their bodies to science. They had tried to sell it, but had been unsuccessful. So now Kerin has a whole little house all to herself, as Jeff says. We put the little orange toy kangeroo in there with her, which made everybody bawl their eyes out. My sister-in-law Bobbi watched Arin in the car, but Elle wanted to be there, and was. The three of us stood like a pyramid rocking, shaking, and crying. (Elle's been like an adult in all this. She and Jeff and I wanted this baby so much. We had *no* ambivalent feelings.) Everyone, including the rabbi, kept telling me I didn't have to go, but I *wanted* to go. And I wanted to help carry the little coffin, with the head facing me, but even *I* didn't realize that I would be resting my head on it, kissing it, clinging to it, and following it into the crypt with my gaze the way a child looks back at a toy in a store window. And I cry as I write this, and bleed, and lactate. Writer that I am, I had thought previously about how I might whisper, "Good-bye, sweetheart; good-bye, little baby," and hoped I wouldn't be too inhibited. I wasn't. And my milk comes yet again—and it's over two days since I've expressed any. . . .

I keep seeing her face; I *want* to keep seeing her face. "She's *such* a cute kid," Jeff says. Her cheeks were round and fat. They said her skin was blue, but I think it was gorgeous: smoothe, not wrinkled, except for the usual peeling fingers. A perfectly shaped head, of course. I keep seeing her little face. I have a photographic memory of her face. (The word "photographic" came out lopsided, because I was, literally, writing through tears.) Her body, too. Such a sweet little baby. She would have fit perfectly in the little French undershirt I bought her, size 3 months, and that little pink Carter's stretch suit, fuzzy and cozy as can be. She never even got to wear any clothes. Not even a diaper. The only thing she ever wore was a little pink ribbon the nurses in the intensive care unit put in her hair, because for some reason they kept forgetting she was a girl and kept calling her "he". Oh, what a little sweetie she was! Sometimes I find myself sending mental signals to her, to wherever she is or isn't, to whatever parallel universes there are in which she pulled through. "Hello, sweetie. Hello, my baby."

Sentimental as all get-out, huh? I'll never get *this* published. Anyway, the following piece of real garbage keeps running through my head:

> *I love little Kerin.*
> *Her skin is so warm.*
> *And if we don't hurt her*
> *She'll do us no harm.*

And the milk runs anew.

Whenever I've just had a baby, I have a tremendous desire

to touch, to get my hands dirty, with the baby as it is, the wet-
ness, the slime, the blood, the meconium (which I used to think
wasn't significant). I want my baby. I want Kerin. Everyone
rushes to touch me, to comfort me. But I want Kerin. Jeff says
everyone understands that and doesn't mind.

I love little Kerin.
Her skin is so warm. . .

Last night I had a dream. (And every night I look forward
to going to sleep because I hope I'll have a good dream.) I
dreamt one of my out-of-this-world nightmare dreams in which
Jeff and I were in this big scary sort-of haunted house and there
were all these sort-of demons in the house. All over the place,
sprawled on the couches and chairs and hanging from the ban-
nisters and chandeliers. Sort-of human demons, having orgies,
sexual and otherwise, all twisting and turning and scary, and for
some reason Jeff and I had to pretend we were going along with
it. I guess so we could eventually conquer the demons. Which
we did. And while Jeff "held down" the demons, I negotiated
with the "chief demon". "All right," he finally asked, "what
do you want?"

I stared significantly. "I want—Kerin," I told him.

"Oh, but that's impossible. . ." he began.

"Don't give me that," I pounced, twisting his arms behind
him like in those detective programs. "You heard me. I want
Kerin."

"Well. . . " his face paled. "I guess that can be arranged."

"That's better," I loosened my grip. "Now, where is she?"

As he was telling me, I awoke. But it made me feel better
for a while.

Not because it gave me an opportunity to vent anger
against someone—I haven't felt much anger yet, against God or
anyone, just grief—and not because I need to feel there must be
some way to get Kerin back (although I do)—but because it expressed a feeling I have, a feeling which I expect to last a long
long time, because it lasted with Arin for something like two
years. See, compared to Kerin, compared to a baby, the rest of
the world's like demons. It's like one big orgy. Like, imagine
having company and sipping tea and conversing about the state
of the union and there's a baby asleep in the next room. Like

my mind's always on the baby. Eight and a half years ago, I used to say, in my lingo, "*Mean*while little Marielle is peacefully sleeping away." I don't know exactly. . . the dream expressed it for me.

A few things I cling to: The first and foremost is my next pregnancy. As soon as possible. As soon as my health permits and as soon as I can conceive. Soon, soon, soon. I can't possibly be more anxious about it than I was about conceiving Elle or Arin but I'm certainly not *less* anxious.

Fears. Fears that I won't ovulate; fears that one or both of us will get killed, or cancer, or sterile. Fears I'll need a hysterectomy, fears that Jeff is too sick, fears that for some reason Jeff will change his mind about having another baby—ya know, Kafkaesque fears.

How soon? we ask each doctor. It gives us something to do. Two months. Three months. Three to six months. Six months. Jeff, with his usual precaution, picks the largest number. I feel I can't bear to wait six months. I feel I can't bear to wait at all. The next baby won't be Kerin but it will be the next baby.

Another thing I cling to: the delivery. Its memory. So much else has intervened so it isn't that strong. But we have a recording. Yes, this time we did it. In fact, Jeff surprised me by recording the whole labor. People advised us not to, but we spent last night and this afternoon listening to it. I'm so glad we've got it down. I want every memory I can get, every souvenir I can get, every tear I can get. It's sad, the labor and after delivery. I didn't remember how serious they felt the situation was. But the delivery itself was fabulous, and I was happy, and the happiness shows. Jeff and I listen to the tape like teenagers listening to records; we smile, sometimes laugh, sometimes cry. We're glad we have it.

Another thing I cling to—the pictures. Jeff took 28. We'll have more pictures of this baby in the first two days than any other. One of her head coming out, several of her being tended to at B—, most of her at Jefferson. She's got a tube in her mouth, and monitors taped all over, but we won't care. We won't care.

I haven't figure out whether or not to be angry. I

haven't yet figured out how to tie it in with the feelings I've always had about God being against me. And I haven't decided how I feel about delivery day being the day after that rejection letter (which ceases to be important to me).

I'm not really angry; I mean this is really a *tragedy*. But then, maybe it's just that I can't bear the thought of God finally *really* crashing down on me. Maybe I'm just shrinking desperately from that thought.

Mostly, though, I'm sad, and it's Kerin I'm thinking of. Her little face, and her feelings. How much did she suffer? Was the extra time in my womb worth it? Wouldn't she have preferred to do dp-dp-dp and play rug-gy with Elle?

A few fantasies I've had which sustain me: One is that I have this very good baby who sleeps all the time, upstairs in the little bassinette, out of the way. I really wouldn't want it that way, but with Elle, my first, I would have. When she was a baby, I used to sometimes sort-of wish that she had died, that I could just lie awake with my postpartum body and think about her birth and not have to get up and change and bathe and worry about her.

Kerin has done some good things for Jeff. First of all, she's made him cry. Secondly, this is the first baby he feels he's really played with and gotten to know at such a young age. Not that he didn't do his share of changing diapers and giving me days off with Elle and Arin. But he admits that he's now learned to enjoy tiny babies. And thirdly, he wants to stay home with the next one. And he's definitely taking a leave—sick or otherwise—next year. (Right now he's on sabbatical.) "With the next one, you're going to have competition," he says. And he won't forget his present mood.

So Kerin has done some good things for Jeff. But she would have done other good things if she had *lived*. As you know, I don't go in for that kind o' crap about God moving in a mysterious way. God doesn't know what's best for Jeff and me, and I'd resent "his" making our decisions for us if "he" did. And, anyway, even if Kerin could do those things for Jeff only by dying, well, then, it's not worth it. We'd rather Jeff keep his hang-ups, if it means keeping Kerin. And Kerin, by the way, is *not* some instrument of God in disguise. She's a little teeny baby, she's Kerin; she's our baby.

For a while, there, I admit I was sort-of getting some small comfort out of my role as chief mourner. But I admitted it, and I didn't feel guilty about it. Because it's as always. I can't have Kerin, so I take what I can get—be it attention, self-pity, or the honor of being chief mourner. I'd much rather have Kerin, sleeping in the bassinette, or crying while I change her, or going dp-dp-dp, or being held and admired by grandparents.

I wanted to give my mother a baby, too. She's had such a hard year, with my father dying, my frank letters to her, and some changes in her friendships. So I wanted so much to give her something nice. When I expressed this feeling to her, new tears appeared in her eyes.

Me to Arin: *Arin, I know I'm in a pretty bad way right now, but if you don't stop making that racket, you're still not gonna like what's gonna happen.*

Me to Elle: *El, just because* I'm *crying doesn't mean* you *have to cry. I mean, don't feel guilty or anything because you're not crying as much as I am. People are different and they react in different ways. And besides—I'm the one who pushed 'er out.*

Writing is really helping to sustain me. What'll I do when the ideas stop?

Me to Arin: *Well, Pokey, I guess you feel a little relieved that you're not gonna be a big brother after all. I mean, maybe you feel just a bit happy that there's no baby after all. But don't get* too *smug; you're only gettin' a repreive!*

Everyone at B— has been calling me. E— and Dr. M— and today this counselor who, she says, is available any time for mothers who have lost their babies. She's very nice, but do I need a counselor? I doubt it, with my writing and Jeff and all. I mean, I consider myself a very well-adjusted person. And I'm not having any trouble crying or anything. Not by a long shot. And speaking of Jeff, why doesn't this counselor call *him* up.

True, I'm the one who pushed 'er out, but he's been affected too. I mean, the whole thing smacks of Nursing Mothers, and doesn't seem terribly feminist. "Is there anything I can do?" asks the counselor. I feel like answering, "Yes, bring Kerin back."

Not "meanwhile little Marielle is peacefully sleeping away," but "meanwhile little Janey Kerin Suzanne is peacefully lying in her grave." Somehow this gives me comfort. Just to think about her existing.

I keep expecting to awaken from this nightmare. Sometimes I *do* have nightmares which seem so damn real, and which go on and on and on. But this one's taking *too* long.

Usually I'm anxious *not* to lose my post-partum figure—I love it so, am so proud of it, take a feminist attitude towards it, like fat liberation. And I *like* bleeding, and stitches hurting, and a flabby stomach, because it all reminds me of the birth.
But this time it's different. I've *got* to get in shape so I can get pregnant again. I've *got* to.

Usually when I wake up, my first reaction is "Damn!"

I try to convince myself that it's being *preg* I live for, and not the actual next birth.

I can do something about my figure, my uterus, my stitches, my bleeding. I can do my post-partum exercises religiously and take all the vitamins I need. But I can't do a damn thing about time. That has to pass, and I have to move alongside it. And be conscious.

Once, around the due date, Elle had said to me in impatience, "If you really wanted to have the baby, you could." Oh, God! that couldn't have been true. I did want to have the baby. I was impatient, too. I was a *little* nervous about how long labor would last, but not *that* nervous.
Yes, lately I've been torturing myself with thoughts like that. *Is* there anything I could have done? Is there anything *they* could have done? Couldn't they have sucked out the

meconium *before* she was born? Couldn't they, or we, have done something? Did we visit her enough in the hospital? If I had talked to her when I was still on the delivery table, could I have made her cry? Oh, if only she had cried after ten minutes, like Elle did! Oh, if only she had lived the week! Then she would be "out of danger". Oh, if we could only divide by 0, we could prove that $1 = 2$, $2 = 3$, and all *sorts* of fantastic things. Too bad we can't divide by 0.

The days will dribble like a leaky faucet. Say, there are 150 of them (before I can get preg). Or 200 (before I *know* I'm preg). Well? So? It's only a day. I can count each one. So far, seven have passed. It'll go faster after awhile. Pretty soon we'll get to 200. I've lived almost 35 years so far; I got through those.

God willing, I'll get through the 200 days. But *is* God willing? I mean, s/he wasn't willing to let Kerin live. *Is* God willing?

My mother's been calling my good friends and telling them what happened. I also asked her to tell them to call and/or visit me *next* week, when I'll need it more. I just wouldn't want visitors now. I mean, as my mother says, this is just so poignant. Two days old. A baby. Labor, delivery, and a baby. I can't let the demons in yet.

Not that we're sitting shiva, and not that I believe in sitting shiva, but now I understand. Why they cover the mirrors, *i.e.*, whenever I'm sad, about *anything*, whenever I've been crying, I always hate to look in the mirror. I feel as though my reflection is mocking me. Especially around the lips.

When I do look in the mirror, though, I see the same kind of face I saw after the other two births. I'm not happy, I'm very sad, but what I see is still a beautiful face with beautiful skin that's chapped from tears but still fresh and shiny from labor and delivery and two days with Kerin. In other words, I'm still proud of being post-partum.

Is that why the baby died? Because I wrote a poem called "Solipsist in Labor"? Did I make the baby jealous? Or, was the *continuity* simply broken? Because, for just one second, I stopped, and therefore the *placenta* stopped? Did my poetry kill my baby? Did solipsism kill my baby? Oh my God, don't you know I was only kidding?

December 30, 1977

I'm no solipsist *now.* No existentialist, either. Never again will I write a solipsist poem, or even a Politics of Motherhood poem. All I care about is baby. Baby, baby. Solipsist or not, I created her. I wouldn't destroy her. Certainly not in the process of creating her. Oh my, oh no, I would never do that. Somebody or something *else* had to have. . .

I keep trying and trying to create her again. But I can't. I just can't. No emotion is stronger or more sincere than baby, baby. Definitely, definitely, I don't own this universe.

January 1, 1978

Yesterday I said, "Jeff, I wish I could just fall asleep and wake up three months from now. Or better yet, a year from now."

Jeff said, "Yeah, you can wake up just as they're saying, 'Okay, now push!'"

That made me burst into a smile, and then into tears. "That's a good one," I said after a while. "I'll write that one down."

Then I said, "That's how it'll *seem* when it happens."

"I know," answered Jeff.

The kids come back today. I am so afraid Elle and I will look at each other and associate and avoid. I don't feel that it's *my* fault, or that *I* have disappointed Elle, but I do feel as though I have been used as an *instrument* for disappointing Elle.

Sometimes I try to convince myself that all the world's a stage, that nothing is real, etc. etc. But I can't. *Everything* is real. *Very* real, for me. After pushing out a baby, *everything* is real. Far, far too real.

I'm afraid to do things that make me forget because then when I come out of it, the reality hits me hard, and I cry hard.

I've cried so many times. Sometimes I wonder whether it really *does* help.

Arin: The whole family's poor 'cause the baby died.
Elle: Arin, we're not poor; we're sad.
Me: Well, we're the *other* kind of poor.

Dr. M—— called again today. Among other things, I had told her that I'm a writer and was writing poems and diary entries about Kerin. So today she asked, "Are you going to bring in the poems when you come for your four-weeks appointment?"

"Sure," I answered. "If you'd like to see them."

"I won't look at them when you're around," she said, " 'cause I'm like you. I get all sentimental and I'd probably burst into tears."

So now, of course, I'm wondering if maybe she'll have some in's for publishing them! In light of Kerin, I don't much care, but still, I'm wondering. Am I a demon, too?

Awful reality thumps. Especially early in the morning. It gets less thump-y in the afternoon—and towards evening I begin to think of sleep. Sweet unconsciousness. Or dreams of Kerin. Also, passing time, passing the time.

But mostly unconsciousness. Or a different *kind* of consciousness.

At night it is *vacuously* true that Kerin is alive and well.

Whaddaya mean, she is not dead, she is only away? Whaddaya think I'm crying about?

Wanna hear something funny? Actually, it turns me ice cold when I think of it. On the morning of Kerin's birth, the morning after that rejection letter, I said to Jeff, "I've decided. I'm not going to make pessimistic comments anymore—ya know, say things like 'And now I bet God's gonna make something go wrong with the baby.' I don't really believe it, anyway, I just do it to beat God to the punch. But so what? So I beat "him" to the punch? So what does *"he"* care?! "He" doesn't mind getting beaten to the punch, if "he" gets what "he" wants. Nope, no more of this nonsense. It's ridiculous; I don't believe in God, anyway. Enough of this nonsense. From now on I'm gonna 'think positive'. And I really *do* have a feeling the baby's gonna be born today or tomorrow. And it's gonna go real fast, and nothing's gonna go wrong. Yup, that's what's gonna happen."

"Good," responded Jeff.

Thinking of that conversation turns my blood ice cold.

I try to think that I was lucky with my first two meconium babies, rather than *un*lucky with the third. But all I know is: *As far as I knew, the probability was that I would have a baby around the house.*

I want so desperately to believe that it was only an accident, and not that God is against me. You know, I read in *The New Age Baby Book* that there are cultures which believe in personal gods—you know, for each person—who stay with that person from birth to death and who do both good *and* bad things to that person. So I'm not the only one.

There must be some truth in it. By that I mean there must be some psychological reason why people feel that way. And I realize that I have the conflicting feelings that (1) God is against me, and (2) God is specifically watching over me, and loving me, and making sure that no *real* harm comes over me.

After what's happened, I don't have feeling (2) any more. But I'm not sure it won't return. Remember, it's a *feeling*. And feeling (1) fills me with dread. Mostly, I wonder: why have I had these feelings? What are they symbolic of?

It's gonna be many, many weeks 'til I can even try to conceive again. Even *try* to *conceive.*

Each day, I've decided, I'm going to accomplish something. I mean something besides writing and getting meals on the table. Even if it's just a little thing. Like writing certain people to tell them what happened. Or sending out one manuscript. Or paying bills. *One* thing. That should help pass the time.

Here are some things to do: Send the rejected "Motherhood" manuscript somewhere else (I have another lead); type up some Kerin-poems; get my other books ready to send out; write my story "The School" (I have the idea, I had it years ago, when Elle started kindergarten, but I haven't been able to write it up satisfactorily. I think I'll try writing it in the style of "The Eternal Baby"); do the chair cushions; make my 4-weeks appointment; read up on health books; help Jeff write *his* story about Kerin, etc., etc. Plus, make plans, appointments, etc.—say, one a week—so the weeks fly by, and maybe the months.

In order to make time pass, I've got to let in the demons. What I really want is Kerin's perfectly shaped head peeking out from the carriage cover.

January 5, 1978

So I do my one thing a day? So?

So while I'm doing it, I'm crying silently, and sometimes not so silently. And my blood runs cold because of the conflict between that thing and Kerin. Because of the demons.

And then, when I'm finished with that one thing, I cry *violently* because, for one, I realize that not much time has passed, only an hour or two. And for another, I realize once again that I will not be Rewarded For My Courage. And along with that comes the realization, the thumping, the thumping of the truth. The eternal-ness of the truth. It will *always* be true. It will *never* stop being true. (Even when I get preg again and even as the new baby cries after being born.) It will *never* stop being true. And it always *was* true; we just didn't know it. We just didn't know it.

The milk is practically gone, so the *animal* part of my longing has probably gone with it. But I guess the animal part isn't a very big part. As an individual, as me, I am that same wild animal, screaming in frantic circles through the forst, searching for my baby. "I want Kerin," I tell each demon.

Some people say that life is temporary, anyway, that everyone dies eventually. Well, so? *Babies* are temporary; I know that from experience; I never aim to make them last forever. It's the *temporary* happiness I expected. It's the temporary happiness I cry over.

Jeff and I both think childlike thoughts. "Well, at least you'll get an extra pregnancy out of the deal" and "Next year when we have the next baby, you'll be thinking 'Kerin would be a toddler by now, but *this* way we get a *newborn* baby right now.' "

If only I had known on the night of the ten-minute-apart contractions. If only I had known. I would have gotten up and *made* her be born. If only I had known. If only. IF only. . . .

That's the thing. I haven't yet accepted it. I just keep thinking about ways it *could* have happened, about happy end-ings. I think of it as something that *almost* happened. I think of it as a narrow escape. And then, when I come back to reality, it thumps hard.

I was in a pretty bad way just a while ago. I wasn't, but I *felt*, completely unable to cope, and as though my nerves were snapping. It was the dinner hour. That seems to be the hardest time. I have no desire to make supper, however simple. It actually *hurts* to make supper. I don't particularly mind *eating*, or sitting around the table with everybody; it's just that initial effort that's so hard. The atmosphere is just so *thick*, like camp when I was a kid. Like a newborn babe myself, I stare at the objects around the room. In a way, my grief takes the form of just plain abstract grief, grief over nothing—grief *qua* grief.

Anyway, I was in a pretty bad way. I began to feel *frightened*, not of not conceiving again, not of anything in the future, but of the *present*. It was, again, an undefined feeling. Frightened *qua* frightened. Perhaps it was hormonal. It's a feeling I get now and then, mostly just before dinner time. It's horrible. It's a nightmare. The feeling, I mean. It's a nightmare. It's not *like* hell—*it's hell itself!*

January 6, 1983

Is it getting better, or are we in between contractions? This morning I didn't cry until ten; later on I found I could feel sad without crying, and this evening I was able to concentrate on a TV program. And I didn't feel frightened today.

I'm not used to this. I'm used to being happy, and acting happy. I feel kind-of disoriented.

I wake up in the middle of the night and think, "I'm not pregnant, and Kerin's dead." Like, when I was an adolescent, I used to wake up and think, "I'm not popular, and there is no God."

It's not fair, I sigh. It's not fair.
Well, *life* isn't fair, they answer, as though disagreeing with me or something.
But we *don't* disagree; we agree.
Life isn't fair, I continue. Life isn't fair.

Whenever Arin acts up, I run off and cry because a *baby* wouldn't purposely act up like that.

Reality doesn't thump anymore. It hangs. Like undigested food. Like a souffle that doesn't rise. Like shit that won't go down the toilet. Reality hangs.

Jeff sucks out my excess milk. Before doing so he holds an' kisses me and tries to dry my tears. "You don't have to give me any foreplay," I say, "*Kerin* wouldn't have."

Last night was bad. First of all, I had some dream about going to some meeting, which was a little bit like the childbirth classes we went to with Arin but also might have had something to do with the Crib Death support group that Dr. M—— and I were talking about yesterday. There really wasn't much to that dream—at least not much that I remember—but when I awoke, I thought, for just a teeny tiny second, that I was still preg. And then, for some reason, I had a horrifying thought:
Suppose, somehow, we miscalculated the conception date?

Or, suppose I made a careless mistake and told them the wrong date? Suppose she wasn't conceived on March 18, but a week earlier? And then, if we had told them the "correct" date, they would have done a stress test on December 18—two weeks after this new due date and maybe they would have noticed something was wrong and induced labor. And then—well, then, it would have been all our fault. A careless mistake, like misplacing one's gloves, could lead to tragedy.

For the longest time I lay awake with my blood frozen, and whispering, actually whispering, "Oh, my God! I'm so frightened. I'm so frightened."

Finally I decided to get up and check the temperature charts. I wasn't sure I could find them, but I did. I quickly looked through, and, thank Goodness, there was no mistake. Kerin was conceived (*i.e.*, I ovulated) on March 17 or 18— probably the 18th. I couldn't possibly have conceived any earlier, certainly not a *week* earlier. Our temperature chart plus Tes-Tape plus cervical mucus all confirmed that.

So I felt much better, almost satisfied, and went back to bed, but not to sleep.

Another little optimistic thing: I just had a baby, and I'm *going* to have a baby.

January 11, 1978

Today we had an appointment with the head of pediatrics at Jefferson, where Kerin was. He was really nice, as everyone at Jefferson has been. He summarized the whole thing for us. Nothing essentially new. It's called "post-maturity", or "post-datism", and I, or Jeff and I, or our babies, have it. It means the placenta and cord cease to function 'way before the labor starts. They don't know why.

And he told us some things about B—. "Look, I'll be honest with you," he up and said, "B— is possibly at fault. For one thing, you should definitely never have been there in the first place. With two late low-birth-rate meconium stained babies. . . They should never have classified you low-risk. . ." And, later on, "Look, I'll come out and say it: If she'd been born here, with our more sophisticated resusitation equipment, she might have lived. . ." My blood rose and fell as he said this, but I'm glad he did.

Talking to this doctor, and to Dr. M———, really helps me. It helps me to accept. It also provides a link with Kerin. And also, as my mother pointed out, it gives me yet another opportunity to talk about the thing that's really on my mind.

"The next baby's coming out early," said Dr. M———, and today Dr. B—— went into some detail. Stress tests, pitocin. . . the whole thing makes me almost happy with anticipation. Something new! I *like* all that attention, I admit it, I like being "closely watched" and fussed over. And most of all, I like (*love*) the idea of the next baby.

I imagine us going to Jefferson for appointments instead of B—. It's so much closer, and it's in a more exciting area, namely, Center City. We could eat lunch out when we go. I imagine the next pregnancy. I have so many associations from the last, and they all make me cry. I imagine us building *new* associations, new memories. Most of all, I imagine the next delivery. We can choose the time of day, Jeff points out, so it can also be not at night. So I can get on the 'phone and scream my happiness to Elle and Arin and grandparents and whoever happens to be my best friends next year. And I imagine how I'll feel before they give me the pitocin. Yes, I'll be scared, but that's not what I'm thinking about. I'm going to feel like a bride on her wedding night. A baby within the hour—that's what I expect.

Once I get going, I get going, and pitocin gets you going.

A baby within the hour! So what if it doesn't work and I have to have a Cesarean? So what if I miss out on pushing? So? It'll be something else. I'll learn the joys of non-natural birth! Of waking up and being told, "You have a beautiful, healthy little boy." You can be sure I'll be ecstatic.

Oh, the happiness that will be mine if only I can wait it out! More accurately, oh, the happiness that will be mine if only God is willing. I go through this all the time. *If* no one gets killed, *if* I conceive, *if* nothing goes wrong, *if...* If time passes, if it doesn't get stuck.

Anyone who believes women were created to bear children must be very unknowledgeable. Look at all the trouble I see. Women who are sterile, women who try for 7 years, women who have three still-births in succession. Accidents of nature are *not* all that rare.

January 12, 1978

The milk dried up two weeks ago. When are the tears gonna dry up?

And where did the milk go? I mean, I hardly expressed any, just a little bit the first two or three days. So where did it go? Where does it go? Maybe the same place Kerin went.

It's not fair. I bite my nails, I used to stutter, I'm mono-gamous, I don't smoke or drink, I'm a married radical feminist, I didn't have dates in high school, and I had all that trouble getting my PhD. It's not fair that I get this, *too*.

God, please, please turn the clock back. Please make me wake up tonight and find I'm still preg., and it's not too late to do the pitocin bit. Please, God, make time go backwards. I promise I won't ask any questions.

This morning I got a 'phone call from someone at the Walt Whitman Poetry Center asking me to do a reading. It's set for June 6. That gives me a *small* lift. For it makes June 6 seem not so far away and it's quite possible I'll be preg by then.

I'm anxious to know what happens when I have my pregnancies close together. In particular, I want to know if the morning sickness situation gets any better. Somehow I suspect it will. I never thought I'd get the chance to find out.

Our trouble, says Dr. B———, is *not* with fertility, not with holding the baby, and not with malformations; it's at the very end. Typical of me.

January 13, 1978

I feel as though my body is saying to me, "Okay, the show's over. Now you can go home." But I can't bring myself to get up and go home.

January 14, 1978

Funny, I often wake up with the memory of a dream plus an awful thought which pounds so strongly—yet seems totally unrelated to the dream.

Now I know why I often think of it as a narrow escape, instead of the reality it is. Because it *was* a narrow escape—the *other* way. We *almost* had a baby. We came so close. We almost had a super-baby. With the vitamins and all. We almost had Kerin. *Almost.*

Sometimes at night I look up and feel a little as though Kerin were looking down on me. I imagine her big. Big like a god. Big like a planet. Big like a monster. And I want her anyway, my baby, even though she's big.

Arin: *Maybe she died 'cause she didn't want to see* me.
Me: *Oh no, Arin. Kerin was very anxious to get to see her big brother. Of course, she knew he might be jealous of her, and she knew he might poke her around a bit, but she also knew he'd be a lot of fun to play with and she* wanted *to see you and Elle very much. It's just that she was sick.*

A friend whom I hardly ever see, but who nonetheless is very close, writes to me, "It's almost springtime."

Elle: *If I could have three wishes, here's what I'd wish: That you'd be pregnant; that Janey would come alive again; and that the nine months would seem like one day to the whole family.*

We're still being brave. We plan trips to the shore this summer, when mommy will be happy again 'cause she'll be preg. We keep on being brave. After I stop bleeding, I tell Elle, she can come in again when I take a bath and then, when I'm preg again, I can show her the colostrium. We just keep on being brave.

The question as to whether or not to share my next pregnancy with the kids seems to be settled. I already am.

The whole family has a sort-of secret rendevouz for some day next January.

Yet one more sense in which women must wait.

Yes, it *has* occured to me that I could resent Kerin for "wasting our time". And no, I don't.

Me: *If I could have three wishes, here's what I'd wish: that Kerin had been born on time; that Kerin had been born on time; and, that Kerin had been born on time.*

Courage, courage; I just had a baby, and I'm *going* to have a baby.

People on the bus don't give me a seat because they don't know I'm post-partum because they don't see any baby.

Arin is *still* a big brother.

January 17, 1978

Not only is it almost springtime, but it's almost *night*time.

And at nighttime, just before I go to sleep, time sort-of loses its meaning, and I feel as though Kerin has just been born, and I feel as though the *next* baby has just been born. It doesn't matter, that it's not now. It doesn't matter. If God were to say to me, "If you get up and walk once around this room, I'll fix it so Kerin was born on time and she's in the bassinette right now"—if God were to give me that opportunity—we'll I'd *almost* say, "I'm too lazy; let me sleep." Almost.

And then, next thing I know, it's the *middle* of the night and I'm up and I'm *not* so drowsy. And things are not so peaceful. Time, *e.g.*, has *every* meaning, and the good times are an eternity away, or in another dimension. And my thoughts are of the "if only" variety. Jeff and I are so knowledgeable; why didn't we know about fetal distress? If only. That B— appointment when my blood pressure went up. The one the week after when it went up higher and my weight went down. And the one still after, the last one, when the blood pressure shot up even more, the weight down even more. I asked them, I *asked* them: was there anything to worry about? Oh no, they answered, nothing to worry about. If only. If only. Or the night of the ten-minute-apart contractions. I was so happy. I didn't *feel* like getting up and walking around. Besides, I've read that Braxton Hicks *can* be regular. You can't stop labor, right?— even if you want to. . .I mean, sure, I was enjoying this little extension of my pregnancy, but not *that* much. It was really more like I was just making the best of things. Like I always do. There's nothing wrong with that—is there? (If only. . . .)

And anyway, suppose it *was* my fault. I mean, suppose the worst. Suppose I did something naughty. Well? So? *I* didn't know. I certainly wouldn't have done it *purposely*. I wouldn't *purposely* kill my baby. I wouldn't *accidentally* kill my baby, either. Search my subconscious well, and you won't find one iota of dislike for my baby. Not even ambivalence.

I don't think I'm really worried that it's my fault; I think I'm worried that people will *think* it's my fault. Or *God* will think it's my fault.

Anyway, when I wake up in the middle of the night, I have to first reconvince myself that there was nothing I could have done, and then, once again, comes the thumping, the pounding, the hanging of reality. The eternal-ness of reality. It isn't the guilt that horrifies me. It's this eternal-ness. As a kid, I had one or two dreams that I had killed my Aunt Faygie. I always woke up relieved and thankful. But it wasn't the guilt, I now realize, that was the nightmare; it was, yes, the eternal-ness of the situation. The irreversibility. I would *always* have killed Faygie. For the rest of my life.

Fears again. Fears that I'll go for my four weeks' appointment and find out I have an infection. Or cancer. Fears that one of us will get killed. Fears that Elle will get killed so I'll never get to give her a baby. Fears.

I write them down in order to beat God to the punch. Crazy. I know it won't matter. It didn't with Kerin. Crazy. I don't *believe* in God. Yet I still sometimes *feel, still*, as though I have my own private God.

What can I say? About the next baby, that is? Only that, if, and mostly *when*, it is humanly possible, I will have another baby. I say so with anger.

Rough beauty. I used to write about it as an adolescent. Weeping mathematicians, and picketers, with chapped hands. Well, that's what childbirth is. Rough beauty.

Actually, that's what *all* beauty is. I mean, babies have guts, flowers have veins, music has amplitude and frequency, and lovers tremble.

"I can imagine how you must have felt after you saw the meconium," my mother said.

"Oh no," I assured her. "I wan't worried about it at all. Elle and Arin had had meconium, too, and besides, when I'm in early labor, I worry about just one thing—namely, how long it's gonna take."

But now I wonder. I mean, I *felt* as though I wasn't worried. But I wonder. In some corner of my mind, I must have been thinking: I'm only *pretending* not to be worried—like the whole world, or a big chunk of it, *pretends* it believes in God. In some corner of my mind, I must have been begging everyone, "Please, please, don't tell me. Not yet. Let me enjoy this birth. Don't take it from me yet."

Wife on TV movie: How long does he have?
Doctor: Two years.
Me to Elle: O! wow! What a long time! I'd *love* to have
Kerin for two years.

If God is punishing me because I think I'm a better mother
than most, then I guess I'll *never* have any more kids, because I
can't help it—I *still* think I'm a better mother than most.

It's not that God had a reason for her dying. It's that *we*
want to *make* there be a reason for her dying.

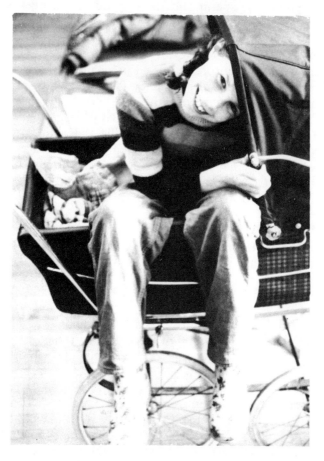

January 19, 1978

Well, I made it through one month. I guess I can make it through three more.

I don't worry about conceiving the baby *after* the next baby. I just worry about conceiving the next baby!

It's all very Kafkaesque. The whole thing—conceiving, carrying, and birth. Will it happen? Suppose? Suppose? Fears. Fears.

Suppose the sperm and the egg are *like* charges; suppose they *repel* each other? I imagine them doing a little dance, a little courtship dance, a little frustration dance. Or suppose the placenta ceases to function *early* in the pregnancy. Or suppose I'm unlucky enough to get a tubal pregnancy, or an abdominal pregnancy, or a cervical pregnancy (some of which necessitate hysterectomy): *i.e.*, suppose the pregnancy is a curse in disguise? Suppose I carry Rosemary's Baby? Or suppose, as occured to me right after having both Elle and Arin, suppose the cervix dilates 10 centimeters and then goes *down* again, before the baby's born, I mean, and I have to go through the whole thing again. Or suppose the head comes out and it's *just* a head, and goes rolling down the aisle?

"Spunky little thing!" said my mother, about Kerin. And now Jeff and I agree that, had she made it, one of her nicknames would have been Spunky.

"We don't know *what* she would have been like," said my mother.

I feel I know *exactly* what she would have been like. Reddish hair, perhaps a few freckles, and the same fattish cheeks; I can just see her in the park playing with the other kids. I see her at age two in that little Mexican embroidered thrift-shop dress. Even more, I see her in that pink Indian gauze dress that I once got on sale for $1. Reddish hair and pink dress. I can just see her skipping about. And I imagine her not having much hair. Like a baby, I guess.

(The telephone rings. I cringe at the loudness. The way a labor contraction makes the baby's heart slow down.)

And I imagine her grown up—say, 21, or my age. This reddish hair again, darkish complexion, tallish—everything *ish*; I don't know why. She'd be calm, not fiery, not exactly like me. And somehow, I imagine that it's at *that* age I get to meet her again. And *I'm* still *this* age (which is 35). She comes over to comfort me. It all reminds me, for some reason, of a poem I once wrote but never perfected, called "Two Women". In it, the present meets the future and I get to meet my future self. And we're a little like mother and daughter. And she tells me all I'm in for—in particular, how long each of my labors is gonna be! It's not the same thing, but somehow it's a little like the above-described meeting with Kerin.

Oh, and another thing about what she would have looked like. She would have looked like a Kerin.

W— called last night. That's the *thing* about most people. The first time you see them after a tragedy, they want you to talk all about it. But by the second time they want you to talk as though it never happened. Anyway, she told me there's an open poetry reading at the Lesbian Center this Saturday night. So maybe I'll go and maybe I won't and maybe I'll read and maybe I won't and maybe I'll read Kerin-poems and maybe I won't. It's all demonish, anyway. I was planning on bringing the baby to these readings, in that little carrier Jeff and I bought. *Meanwhile* little Kerin would have been peacefully sleeping away.

Another fear: That I'll have a false pregnancy. Then it'll waste even *more* time.

Now, I know that I don't "intensely desire" to be *falsely* pregnant. And I know that, even deep down in my subconscious, I'd rather wait another three months and get *really* preg than get falsely preg right now.

But I'm afraid God *thinks* I'm neurotic enough to have a false pregnancy, and I'm afraid he'll make me have one.

We just had the typewriter fixed. Now I can pass the time typing up my next few books, and trying to get them published. Will *this* count as one of those books?

I realize that, for me, God is just whatever it is that causes my own powerlessness. That's why, for me, God is a "he"—and that's why I hate and fear him so.

I used to tell God that if he dared touch any of my children, I'd kill him. Somehow, I seethed, I'd kill him. Now I know I can't. Not even somehow.

"If this is a test," said my mother three weeks ago, "then I must say you've passed with flying colors."
"It isn't over yet," I answered.

Also, if this is a test, then why doesn't God punish me *after* I've failed it, rather than before?

In one of my unperfected Politics of Motherhood "run-on" poems, I wrote *"Just because God meant for mothers to instruct their children in the ways of the world doesn't mean God* helps *mothers instruct their children in the ways of the world"* (*e.g.* He purposely makes the light turn red, just as soon as the mother says, 'Okay, you can cross now'.")
Well, *now* I write: Just because God intended women to exist solely to create children, doesn't mean God intended women to *enjoy* creating children.

Years ago, I had this dream which I considered feminist. I dreamt that there were these two women who had been reduced in size and encased in glass. They were alive and conscious, but they couldn't move. They couldn't breathe, either, but then they didn't *need* to breathe. Still, it was scary, not being able to breathe. The main thing is, the women were completely helpless, and couldn't even *try* to convince the people to let them go. Was that dream a premonition of Kerin? and what she went through?

January 21, 1978

Oh now, see? See what I've done! What a naughty girl I've been! First I tell everybody I'm having a baby, and then I put out my hands and go, "Ha! ha! fooledja!" Naughty, naughty.

Why do I feel so anxious about conceiving? Well, it's a little like waiting for a bus. Once it comes, at least you're on your way. At least you're getting closer and closer to your goal. This way it's just a stand-still.

I know I shouldn't feel this way but how can I stop? And if I *do* stop, maybe I'll *forget* to have another baby. Or maybe God will think, Okay, she's okay; now I can make things such that she can't have another baby.

I'm scared stiff. I'm scared I won't conceive because sub-consciously I feel guilty about not stopping at two. Or about having more kids than my mother had. Or about my body killing Kerin. As I keep saying, I *don't* feel guilty about any of these; I'm just afraid psychologists will *think* I feel guilty *if* it turns out that I can't conceive, and that will somehow *justify* God's not letting me conceive.

I always make the best of things. But there have to be things to make the best of.

January 23, 1978

Actually, it's not that I'm good at making the best of *bad* things; I'm just good at making the best of *good* things. As I wrote in my poem "Ode to Myself", the day after having Arin, I am "the one who makes beautiful things even more beautiful." I sort-of don't know what to *do* with an *ugly* thing. I feel disoriented.

Arin: *I* know how to get mommy to stop crying—give her a present *every* day.

Me: Arin, presents don't make me happy when I'm *sad*; they only make me happy when I'm happy.

PhD in math. Writer, artist, thrift shopper. So well organized; the one time my wallet got stolen, I got it back. —— If I'm so smart, why couldn't I save my baby? Why did I not know it was suffocating—right inside of me? Why didn't I know? Every time it moved so vigorously and desperately, I hugged it and grinned. As Bettelheim says, love is not enough.

Jeff and I were so careful. Vitamins, Adelle Davis, books. And then, of course, we *knew* we couldn't control *everything*; we *knew* about "the best laid plans of mice and men." We knew. I don't see why God had to make this happen to teach us.

January 25, 1978

Two whole days without feeling frightened or horribly low. Is it getting better, or are we in the expulsive stage—when the intervals between contractions get longer but the contractions themselves are impossible? Well, is it getting better, or are we in the expulsive stage?

When I say, or think, "we," as in the above paragraph, I realize that the other part of the "we" is another me. I think of a line from a poem of mine, "I am super-imposed upon myself."

As I told Dr. M—, like anyone who's just had a baby, I want to talk baby-talk. That's another reason for joining one of those support groups.

But suppose I join for the purpose of getting convinced it's not my fault? And suppose they all turn out to think it *is* my fault?

January 27, 1978

Four-week's appointment over (at five weeks, as usual!) I'm in great shape, and Dr. M— says I can get pregnant in two more months. But then Jeff said, "We were thinking, three," and then she said, "Well, I guess there'd be less risk of an early loss at three," so we're back to three.

We also gave her copies of my poems (most of them first drafts) and showed her the letter we wrote to Dr. F— (the main doctor in charge at B—). The letter criticized their policy of being so casual when diagnosing mothers as low-risk, and pointed out that low-risk $\neq$ no-risk. It also denounced the spacing of appointments more than two weeks apart during the last months (and beyond) and the failure to do stress tests even after two weeks overdue. It ended with a plea: "Please, please worry a little more. Please, please, be careful." Dr. M— looked as though she was about to burst into tears.

Arin: I was the best baby. I was the only one that came out crying. And then I breathed. And I breathed and I breathed and I just kept on breathing.

Maybe one of the reasons women love to give birth is that it gives them a chance to relive their own birth traumas.

Yes, I probably *do* believe in birth trauma now.

January 29, 1978

Nowadays, when reality strikes, it doesn't thump or hang; it howls. Like a winter wind. Like a Shakespearean tragedy. When I think about what Kerin went through, reality howls.

Now, if Kerin had lived, it would still bother me, what she went through. But then at least I could comfort her.

I wish I could hibernate this winter. My life is good; I have a good husband, two good children, a good house, a good part-time job. I have a good life. But you see, I've been half-way to heaven. So I know what life *can* be. And I'm not willing to settle for less. I don't know what I'll do if I have to.

It's all so Kafkaesque. *Will* time pass? Will I ovulate? Will I conceive? Will the uterus, the placenta, the cord—will it all do what it's supposed to do? Will whoever's in charge of diluting the pitocen dilute it enough? Or will that person, for some reason, take a disliking to me?

It's all so Kafkaesque. What comes out? Can the monitor and the ultrasound and the oxytocin challenge test and the urine test all come out negative and still the baby be born dead? Can the monitor beep 158 beats a minute all through the pushing, then 0 at birth? Can the Mean Value Theorem fail, in my case?

It's all so Kafkaesque. What comes out? A baby, or a pulsating mass of flesh? What comes out? A baby or a giant insect?

I used to think that such thoughts meant life was meaningless. Now I realize it's just the opposite.

February 3, 1978

Not only are we into February, but it's February *3*—not February 1. And yes, of *course* I realize Feb. is the shortest month, and that it's not leap year.

I've come to realize that, by "we", I *don't* mean me plus another me. I mean me plus a whole *chorus* of mes. All rooting for *this* me.

We bought two textbooks on obstetrics, plus a book on ultrasound. We joked about taking a year off and going to medical school. We joke about our plans for the next baby. We exaggerate. I'm gonna walk around with a stethoscope in my ears, the other end scotch-taped to my belly. On the bus, people are gonna say, "Your first, dear?" And then we're gonna buy a portable fetal monitoring machine, and I'll be a nervous wreck the entire nine-months; I won't take my eyes off that machine. Or maybe I'll even buy a portable ultrasound, or a portable intensive care unit just in case the baby gets born by surprise. I've actually burst out laughing at this.

And then there's another level on which I'm not surprised. I mean, when I think back to that initial meconium, I realize that women live in fear of what they're gonna find in their pants when they go to the bathroom.

Also, I usta have this thing about my long, irregular menstrual cycles. I somehow associated it with my not having dates in high school. But I overcame it; I mean, I never reached the stage where I felt inadequate because of those long irregular cycles. And of course, I just assumed my babies would also be late, and didn't feel there was anything wrong in that.

So now I just *know* that my long irregular cycles have something to do with what happened. Which means that my not having dates in high school has something to do with what happened. Which means that I, the *me* in me, the me I've learned to love, killed Kerin.

So Wednesday night I taught that Math Anxiety Clinic at Temple. As usual, I made the first session into what I call the workshop "runaround". Everybody got a chance to talk about math and math anxiety in her/his life. I was surprised at my ability and willingness to get into it. Every once in a while Kerin would flash through my mind, and I would mentally apologize for becoming a demon, explaining that it was necessary, otherwise the next baby would wind up getting a crazy woman for a mother. And also, I kept thinking how, when it came to be my turn, I would probably tell them about what happened to me, and I was a little nervous about that. And then when it did come to be my turn, I did tell them. I said that what I was about to say was very hard for me, and it didn't have anything to do with math or math anxiety but I usually feel friendly towards the people in the workshop and this was no exception and I felt they should know—I recently had my first tragedy—blah blah blah—and so if I ever suddenly started to cry or act irritable or inattentive, that would be why—and my face felt all red and my voice got all weepy and the eight faces looked so sympathetic—I especially remember the man's— and one woman waited for me to finish talking and then said, "The same thing happened to me."

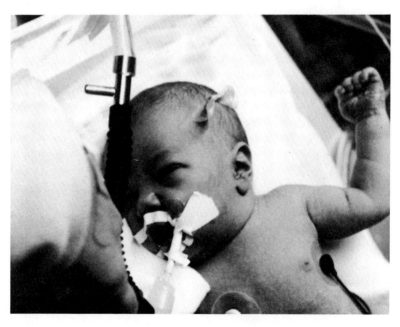

Kerin

People probably think I'm getting better because it's all fading from my mind. But that's not it at all. I'm getting better because there's getting to be less and less time I have to wait before getting preg again.

I just feel so funny *not* being preg. I almost feel as though I *am* preg. I don't know. . . it's like I want people on the streets to know I'm a baby-person.

Yes, I feel as though I *am* preg. And, actually, I am. *Twice* preg. Eleven months' preg with Kerin and minus-two months' preg with the next baby. And that's why I have to keep in good shape—take my vitamins and all—and that's why I sometimes get the feeling that people on the street *do* know. Like, when I'm walking along Chestnut Street, even without the kids, they sort-of smile at me, as though they somehow know I'm poetically preg.

In the middle of the night, if I'm awake, I stare at where the bassinette would be. It seems as though I've wandered into the wrong parallel universe and am trying to find my way back.

Yes, I *am* preg—eleven months' preg and minus two months' preg. I just had a baby and I'm going to have a baby. And yes, it *is* a little like carrying twins.

February 13, 1978

It keeps being true and it keeps being true and it keeps being true. It happened and it happened and it happened. It happened to *us* and it happened to *us* and it happened to *us*.

I was hoping that by the time we got to *that* stage, I'd be preg.

I find that I hesitate to write because I'm afraid God will think, 'Gee, she's really good at writing about that subject; maybe I'll make it happen again so she can write some more."

On the other hand, if I write it all out, then God might think, "There's nothing left for her to write, so there's no point in making it happen again. In fact, what we need are some breast-feeding poems."

Forgetting about God, I'm afraid to write too much because then, if it does happen again, I won't even be able to write about it. I just won't, that's all. What more would there be to say?

They say babies tie you down. But I know I'd get a lot more accomplished if the baby was here.

Arin's fifth birthday is June 23. I worry that it's too soon, that Arin's getting too big too soon. And yet, since it's possible that I'll be preg by then, I worry that it's not soon *enough*. Currazy.

Talking to other people to whom it's also happened, about *it*, keeps me sane because it lets me know that I'm not the only one, that it's a chance thing, that I wasn't specially chosen. It keeps me from being self-centered.

But then *afterward, after I've just talked to that someone,* I get depressed all over again. Because then I'm thrust back into the normal everyday world where babies are born and don't die, and I realize that it really *is* an unusual thing, that I really *was* unlucky, and maybe I really *was* chosen, and that maybe they form groups like UNITE just to make it *seem* as though it's not so terrible, that it happens to a lot of people. Maybe they form these groups just to keep us quiet, to keep us out of the streets, out of their way.

I mean, you could take all the people of *any* class and put them together and then these people would seem perfectly normal. And they'd all say, "See? I'm not the only one." Like, even if there were ten people in the whole world in that group, if they all got together in one room, they'd feel typical and un-alone. I mean, maybe it's political. It's sort-of as though these groups prevent me from being self-centered and going crazy by making it seem as though babies dying is the norm. But maybe I *should* be self-centered and maybe I *should* go crazy because babies dying *isn't* the norm. Well, it isn't. The infant mortality rate is 2%. And I haven't had 50 children. And among non-smokers who eat natural foods and have natural births it must be much less (I don't mean to sound superior, but that is true). The infant mortality rate is 2%—not 100%. Only in UNITE is it 100%. I don't know. . . When I go back to the regular world, I feel depressed and self-centered. And I wonder *Why me?* It strikes me again that it happened. It actually happened. And I can't stand it.

February 16, 1978

Okay, 12 more days, and Feb. will be over. Then we're into March and it wouldn't be so terrible if I conceived then. I
mean, it *sounds* good. Even if it were March 1. It would *seem*
like 3 months. Dr. B— put us in contact with an obstetrician
named Dr. W— and we're going over to meet him this coming
Monday, which is the 20th, when Feb. will really be almost
over. And the 20th is almost here. Also, Martha invited us to
her kids' birthday party, which is on the 26th, and before ya
know it, it'll be here. That's another sense in which Feb. is almost over.

Yup, women were born to wait, it seems, born to wait.
Wait to ovulate when they want to get preg. Wait for their periods when they don't. As I said in a poem, "maybe biology *is*
destiny. But that doesn't make it right."

Martha told her friend Eileen about what happened and
she told me that they both agreed that I was the one who least
deserved it. But rather than bolster me up, it made me feel
more depressed. Because it just confirms my feeling of the un-
fairness of the whole thing. It just makes me angrier. And
sadder. So I don't know what's worse—feeling that I deserved
it, or feeling that I *didn't* deserve it.

I sooo want a baby; I am as into babies as some people are
into sex. It might even be my downfall. I don't know; its as
though God knew I wouldn't let babies run my life, so he gives
me *no* babies (this time—anway).

Because of the no-baby, this year (well, at least the few
months before I can get preg again) is going to be a waste. I
have no interest in writing about anything other than babies. I
have no interest in poetry readings, sewing, feminism, even
math. *Even* thrift shopping. And politically, I'm a wreck. I
mean, babies have always died, and I always knew it; why is it
that only *now* I feel I can't live with that knowledge? How
ethnocentric, how nationalistic can I get? Yes, babies don't do
me in because I've discovered the Politics of Motherhood, so
God gave me *no*-baby. I've got babies figured out, so God gives
me no-baby. I know that's all nonsense, but it's how I feel.

And also—well, ya know about the Bible and how woman

is supposed to "travileth in pain" (ya know, the natural child-birth woman)? And how some of the religious women in this movement say the Bible doesn't mean *bearing* children; it means *rearing* children. And ya know how *this* woman refuses to even *rear* children in pain? Well, I feel as though God's saying, "Okay, woman, you refuse to both bear and rear children in pain? Okay, so I won't let you bear or rear children at all." In other words, I feel that God doesn't like the Politics of Mother-hood very much.

In other words, somebody up there doesn't like me.

Well, why should I *expect* somebody up there to like me? Why should I expect to be liked by those in power? Why did I ever think I *would* be? I never was *before*. I wasn't popular in high school, Wesleyan gave me all that trouble with my PhD, and nobody's ever given me a really decent job. And S.E. Press didn't want my motherhood book. So come on now; I didn't *really* expect God to *like* me?

All this is silly, of course. I met Jeff when I was 15. I have what everyone I know wants—a good relationship. I've had it for 17 years, so even if Jeff dies (that's the only way it could end), I still would have had it for a long time. I mean, I did just happen to meet Jeff. So in that respect God *does* like me. Plus, of course, I have two living children.

No, of course, it's not a question of whether or not some-body up there likes me; it's just chance. And the post-datism is *not* connected to the long irregular cycles; the doctors said so. No, it's just chance. It just *happens* to seem to correlate with my past. And probably, no matter *how* it happened, I would (especially being a writer) find *some* correlation with my past.

Here's another way I feel: again, this mad passionate desire for a baby could be my undoing. Until I'm preg, *e.g.*, I won't be able to concentrate on anything else. And I'll do almost any-thing to get preg, *e.g.*, even if I didn't love Jeff, "I'd stay with him. Just to have someone to give me a baby."

Gone is my pride. I'll do anything God wants me to do, even if I don't agree with him. On the streets, *e.g.*, I smile at old ladies, open doors for people, say "excuse me" when I bump into anyone, and am the epitome of patience while wait-ing in line at Acme. I don't really believe these things are terribly important, and I think that, under the circumstances, my failure to do them would be understandable, but I'm determined to be a good girl. I'm scared stiff; I'll do anything, anything, so God doesn't punish me again.

That's how it feels, anyway. I'm scared stiff. Yep, I've really got the fear o' the Lord in me. I now know what the fear o' the Lord *feels* like. I'll do anything the Lord wants. Anything. The trouble is: I don't *know* what he wants. How can I know? He doesn't tell me, and I don't have a very good sense of ESP. How can I possibly know?

I try to guess. Does he want me to grieve profusely, or doesn't he? If I grieve profusely, then maybe he'll say I'm pitying myself. But if I don't, then he could say I'm running away from it. If I do, he could say, "*I'll* give you something to cry about." (Like not being able to have another baby or Jeff getting killed.) On the other hand, if I don't, he could think (or pretend to think) I don't love Kerin enough.

And should I talk to everyone about our plans to have another baby? If I do, then God could think that's silly; how can I be *sure* I'm going to have another baby? If I don't, then he could accuse me of not being honest.

In particular, should we talk to the *kids* about our plans for the next baby? If I do, God might think that's bad psychologically, because how will it affect the kids if something happens with that baby, too? If I don't, then God might also think *that's* bad psychologically, because the kids will wonder what's on our minds.

What does God want? If I only knew, I would oblige, so anxious am I to have another baby.

Again, that's how I *feel*. And okay, so: I don't know, can't possibly know, what God believes. But I *do* know what *I* believe. And so I grieve a whole lot, but laugh when I feel like it, and I do talk to everyone, especially the kids, about the next baby. I do what I always do—namely, what I believe in.

But I'm in a precarious position, and I know it.

The greatest fear is that I won't ovulate. The greatest fear by far. I imagine the egg trying to break away, like in my poem ("Doors trying to escape their hinges"). I imagine the egg tied to a rubber band, so it *almost* escapes, so it *does* escape, but is pulled back by the rubber band. (Rubber bands seem to be fascinating symbols). I mean, suppose I never ovulate again? Or suppose it takes a year to ovulate? If I knew *how* to ovulate I would, but I don't know how. I don't know how.

So yesterday, around 7:00 p.m., I said, "Okay, I've had enough of it being Feb. 20. Now I'm ready for it to be Feb. 21."

Then, "Yes, I'm ready to go to bed and wake up and find that it's Feb. 21. Or better yet, *March* 21."

Now I know the meaning of the following joke:
"*What's today?*"
"*The 21st.*"
"*The 21st?*"
"*Yep. All day.*"

All day. All. Day. Ten o'clock. Eleven o'clock. Twelve o'clock. All the way to ten o'clock, again. Like I said, all day.

I read in natural childbirth books all about the horrors of medicated birth. The woman gets put in a wheelchair, says good-bye to her husband, gets a paracervical block, then in general, wakes up to be told she had a girl, is groggy for the next few days, gets put in a wheelchair again before her husband picks her up to take her and the baby home. Oh, how I wish I could have been that woman!

Yes, it will be my downfall. I adore birth in any form. I adore pregnancy, I adore birth, I adore babies. I am sooo proud of my births, all three of them. I am proud to be a multipara, proud to be gravida 3. Proud to tell any doctor my obstetrical history. I know it wouldn't be my fault if I were sterile, but I'm sooo glad I'm not. (I might be proud of it if I were.) I'm proud of my short labors and I guess I'd be just as proud if my labors were long. If I have a Cesarean next time, I'll be proud of that.

It's such a big thing in my life. *This* part of my life, anyway. I know it has to end sometime, but not now. Please, God, not now. I don't mind being old, but I do mind being *too* old to have a baby. I suppose eventually I'll be satisfied. Eventually I will have had enough. I suppose. But not yet. Please, God, not yet.

February 23, 1978

Yesterday I said to Jeff, "I'm in touch with my body, but my body's not in touch with me." Then I exclaimed, "Hey, that's a good one! I'm gonna go write that one down."

Although I didn't really talk all that much at the UNITE meeting, I did get my two cents in about how I think of pregnancy as a thing in itself, that I'd get pregnant even if I knew the baby was gonna die in the end, that having the baby with you for that period of time was nice, too. Of course, I added, my pregnancies and deliveries are easy, so I can afford to say that. I have nothing to lose by being pregnant.

Some of the women there were already preg again, and others were thinking about it. But I was the only one who *said* I was gonna get preg just as soon as possible, and the sooner the better.

"So I take it you're optimistic," said the UNITE psychologist.

'Yes I am," I responded. "But, of course, I can afford to be optimistic. Ya know, I have two healthy children and they know what to do about my problem so there's no reason to suspect I can't have more."

I was, in a sense, apologizing for being optimistic. I had "optimistic-guilt"! Sort-of like white-guilt.

Oh, God, don't punish me for being optimistic, or for thinking a lot of myself for being optimistic. (Crazy; all this is crazy.)

But God, I *have* to be optimistic, because it'll be bad for the next baby if I'm not. I've read that tension can be transmitted through the placenta, and also the next baby will need my love and confidence, whether it lives or not. Besides, I *do* have every reason to be optimistic. And I *want* to be optimistic.

I'll *never* ov; I just know it. I'll be one of those women who take a year to ov. Yer derned tootin' my body isn't in touch with me. It thinks I don't need a baby; it thinks I already have a baby. It doesn't know my baby is dead; all it knows is what goes on inside it. True, it should realize it's not lactating, but maybe it doesn't. Maybe it's stupid. A smart mind in a stupid body. Maybe that's my curse.

I can *so* "emotionally handle a pregnancy". I can *so* go through "the grief process" and the creation-process at the same time. But maybe my body is the same kind of dunce as some psychiatrists. Maybe my body is on *their* side.

Yeah, whaddaya mean, can I "emotionally handle a pregnancy"? Just try me; *i.e.*, give me a chance—dammit! give me a chance. And, anyway, I can much better emotionally handle a pregnancy than a *non*-pregnancy. And also, the sooner I get preg, the less time there'll be for my fears to build up.

About this "grief process", I'm sick and tired of it. I'm sick and tired of being sad *all* the time. Maybe I'm rushing through life, as I rush through labor, but I'm ready to get on with it. It's time to get preg. It *was* time to get preg the minute L'il Spunky died. Maybe the psychiatrists, God, and my body don't believe that's healthy, but I do. And, if I'm permitted, I'm going to act on it. I'm going to have another baby just as soon as possible. If God wants to stop me, he can. But the first ov after March 22, I'm getting preg. That's it. I need a little heartbeat in my uterus and, if and when possible, I intend to get it.

Eileen says I have to relax. Well, I think I *am* relaxed, but so what if I'm not? Why should I not ov just because I *want* to ov? It just doesn't make sense; why should my body play hard-to- get?

In other words, in order to ov, I have to convince myself that I don't *want* to ov. Crazy. I have to convince myself that I don't give a damn. But how can I do that? I *know* I want to ov. "To thyself be true," they say, and I know no other way. That's supposed to be good, healthy, etc.; so why am I being punished for it?

Damn it! I've got this great healthy attitude about wanting like mad to get preg again, but I *can't* get preg if I don't ov.

And Feb 26 and Feb 26 and Feb 26.

Okay, now I get the idea. Yeah, yeah, I get the idea. It keeps on being like this 'til I go crazy from boredom if nothing else. So c'mon, let's get on with it.

Grief process, schmief process, it's time to get preg. I guess I'm one of those women who, if I weren't monogamous for all time, and if Jeff got killed, I'd be looking around for someone else right away. "Okay, now," is what I'd be thinking. "I know I'm gonna wind up finding someone else, so I might as well go right ahead and do it! Why postpone it? Why be miserable? I might as well at least be *happy* while I'm going through the grief process."

But I *am* monogamous for all time, so that's not what I would do. But babies are different. I'm not monogamous when it comes to babies. I can mourn one baby while loving another. Like the woman in "Sumer of '42", who, upon learning that her husband had been killed in the war, finds comfort in the arms of a fifteen-year-old kid. I can find comfort in another baby.

Maybe that's one reason I love childbearing so much. Maybe it gives me a chance to keep experiencing new loves. I don't think that's true, but it's a thought.

Anyway—okay, okay, I get the idea. Feb. 26. And now that I've mastered Feb 26, let's move on to Feb. 27.

I feel as though God, knowing (from observation) that I can be a feminist mother, has decided to do this to me because he knows that's the only way to knock me down. Like the boss trying to break up the union.

Funny, but I haven't really voiced my anger yet. I've cried plenty, and spoken about how I feel, but I haven't really had a temper tantrum yet. Funny, I always used to say that if anything *really* bad ever happened to me, I'd probably take it quite calmly. And I guess I was right. There were two reasons, I think, for this: (1) I now know, as I never knew before, that temper tantrums do no good, and (2) I've *already* had so many temper tantrums, so I know that a temper tantrum over *this* would have been a doozer, and I know that I probably couldn't top the temper tantrums I've had in the past. In other words, a temper tantrum wouldn't adequately express my feelings, since I've already had so many of them over minor matters.

February 28, 1978

I had a good conversation with Dee this morning. When I called her, *she* had been crying, so I hung up saying I'd call back later. So then *she* called me back and we talked for about two hours. *Her* trouble is that she's got a lesbian custody case on her hands. Her ex-husband's been working up to it for a while, and now it seems he means business. The kid in question is 12-year-old Kippy. Anyway, Dee fulfilled my needs. She listened and we talked. In particular, she assured me that I'd have another baby (and told me about her ex-sister-in-law, who, at her six weeks' check-up, was told she was preg!) We talked about guilt, depression, all kinds of things. Analyzed things, laughed. I assured her I didn't feel *obligated* to be depressed. Yep, Dee's friendship has lasted well over the years. And today she saved me from a day of gloom.

March 2, 1978

Coming in like a lion, and whether or not it will go out like a lamb depends on what my innards decide to do.

For some reason I want to cease essentially all activity until I get preg. Just cook, write, go grocery shopping, wash clothes, and do only what's absolutely necessary. Be a schlepp. For some reason, that's what I feel I want and need. I'm not sure why that is. Maybe it's because I want to get the sadness out of my system. Maybe it's because I've never been a schlepp fore and I want to try it out. Maybe I need to have a marked period of mourning. Maybe I'm just lazy. I don't know. But I want to postpone life until I get preg.

And I feel as though God is saying, "Oh, *no* ya don't! Yer not gettin' off *that* easy! *You* have to show *me* that you can be brave and accomplish things *before* you get preg. *Then* I'll let you get preg. (Maybe.)"

Why do I feel this? Because I feel that the world, that part of the world that has power, has a different opinion of me, psychologically, from what I do. And I feel that, although *I'm* right, *it* will prevail. In other words, as usual, I feel my own powerlessness.

March 4, 1978

Thrift shops, poetry readings, sewing—it was all simply a celebration of my happiness. Now I can bear none of it.

And I used to think that maybe, Deep Down Inside, the above were an Escape. (I mean, since so many psychiatrists would say that, I thought maybe they were right.) Now I *know* otherwise.

One of the things that gets me mad is that, if Kerin were born on the due date, Dec. 11, instead of Dec. 22, I'd have less time to wait to ovulate. Of course, if she'd been born on Dec. 11, I wouldn't have to be going through all this in the first place. But it makes me mad anyway. Like adding insult to injury.

I imagine myself being preg. And I feel all happy and not worried at all. "But what about placenta previa, or cervical pregnancies?" I remind myself.

"Nah, that won't happen to *me*," I answer.

Just like the good ol' days. Nothing *really* bad happens to me.

As long as I have L'il Fetus inside me, I'll feel safe.

Yer darn tootin' I feel sorry for myself. And I feel sorry for anyone else who goes through this, too.

In the past, just after I had both Elle and Arin, I'd think,

"Gee, some women go through labor and then their babies die. Now I know God has done some pretty cruel things in his day, but somehow that seems the cruelest. To do that to a woman fresh from labor. And to kill a baby."

I guess part of the reason I thought that was to protect myself from it happening to *me*. I don't know. . . I guess I thought if I *didn't* think that, God would decide to make it happen to me so I could *learn*. I don't know. . . And I guess what must've happened was: either God *forgot* what I'd thought, or else he believes I didn't think *enough*.

To think that just a few months ago I used to believe that, no matter what happened, I could live and be happy, as long as I had My Self. Well, I don't believe that anymore. Because I've been halfway to heaven. And even if and when the memory fades, I'll still remember that there *was* a heaven. That it **was**.

And another thing: having just been thrust out of heaven, I can tell you this: Nothing—nothing—is as intense as baby, baby. Not math, not the night, not my early childhood—nothing. Compared to baby, baby, even my nostalgia-poems and my insomnia-poems and my general-anesthesia-poems, and, yes, even my baby-poems are superficial as a cocktail party. Yes, even *they're* demonish. I know that sounds crazy, and it'll probably sound crazy to *me*, too, sometime in the future, but it is definitely true. I've just been there and I know.

March 11, 1978

And one more thing: whenever I hear about something that's supposed to be Nirvana—whether it be something possible like LSD or something impossible like heaven—well, I would *rather* have baby, baby, than any of these things. In other words, I would rather have baby, baby, than heaven itself. I want baby, baby, more than I ever wanted anything, except, probably, when I was an adolescent, to fall in love. I want baby, baby, more than I wanted that PhD, and more than I wanted to get a book published.

In fact, it appears I am going to get that math-poetry book published, and I do give *part* of a damn, but not a very big part. "The Weirdest Is the Sphere." By Marion Cohen. Seven Woods Press. First publisher of Susan Fromberg Schaeffer. I should be thrilled. I've wanted it for so long; I've waited so long. At least I *thought* it was waiting. Now that I'm waiting for baby, baby, I realize that I wasn't waiting at all. Not with that hour-by-hour, day-by-day, it-has-to-be-now kind of desperation. No, I wasn't waiting then at all; *e.g.*, I had whole days, whole weeks, when I didn't think about it at all. I'd go thrift-shopping, take the kids to the movies, happy and willing to wait as long as I had to. But not so with baby, baby.

I already have two babies—three, really—on my world line. But it's not on my world line I want baby, baby; it's now. "Be here now," says Guru Ram Dass. Well, this whole Kerin-thing had made me realize that I usually *do* "be here now" and that's one of the reasons I'm so disoriented. I'm not *used* to rushing time onward. In other words, in many respects, being well-adjusted makes things *worse*.

Jeff and I read that PABA and manganese help stimulate the pituatary gland, which helps stimulate ovulation. So I've started taking 3 tablets a day. Will it help? As Jeff says, it can't hurt.

I try to be optimistic. Just to avoid being nervous. Each morning, if the Tes-Tape is a little darker, or the temperature a little lower, or a little higher, or the mucus a little wetter, if anything at all, I get optimistic. Not excited, just optimistic. Or rather, not pessimistic. Spinnbarkeit means the mucus can be stretched. It's supposed to happen around ov-time. I'd recognize it without even trying to stretch. Mittelschmerz is a pain "felt in the lower abdomen, often on the right side, non-radiating.' *That* I *wouldn't* recognize. Very often, more than once a month, I get pains in the lower abdomen, or the right side, and non-radiating. Muscle twinges, gas pains, I don't know. I'm just not one of the "15% of all women" who "get well-defined Mittelschmerz."

Anyway, the problem is not to *recognize* the ov. It's to ov, period. Or rather, to ov with *no* period.

Yep, someday all this is gonna be *funny*. I mean, it *will* have its element of humor. Only if I eventually get preg, though.

Come on, Spinnbarkeit—start spinnen! Come on, Mittel-schmerz—start schmerzen!

Come on, ov—why are you so late?!

I just remembered that I had planned to dedicate my book to L'il Kerin. Very slightly, I hesitate. Because: whenever I read a dedication that says something like "to the memory of" so-and-so, or whenever the author claims she wants to "preserve the memory of so-and-so," well, I always feel skeptical. I feel that the author's really just *using* so-and-so to make her book sadder or something. I don't know. I don't *think* it's just pro-jecting. The feeling is similar to, but not the same as, when authors admit they got the idea from something so-and-so said, but they don't mention so-and-so's name. As if they're afraid so-and-so might get the credit.

So I'm afraid I might be using Kerin in some way, to get attention or something. Would there be any truth in this? I really do want L'il Kerin to be remembered. And I do want everyone to know that I was preg and gave birth 3 times, not twice. (Or rather $n + 1$ times, not n- - hoping $n > 2$).

Jeff says, "See ya later, ovulater!"

March 16, 1978

At first I tried to *will* myself to ov. I carefully studied a diagram of the ovaries and then imagined, as hard as I could, the whole thing happening. But then I read somewhere that the *pituitary* gland stimulates the ovaries, and I thought, "Ah, forget it! The whole thing's much too complicated. You don't simply ov; it's all tied in with the pituitary gland. It's a whole network. I couldn't possibly figure it out. I'll just have to wait 'til it happens by itself."

Oh, I'm smart, all right—just not smart enough. Not smart enough to ov, and not smart enough to save Kerin. As I said in my one-line poem, my "tidbit", "God gave me a gift of talent. But he tied it with Gordian knots."

Anyway, March 16. March 16. When I wake up tomorrow it'll be March 17. And then, of course, the next day, the probable anniversary of Kerin's conception. When I think of my life around that time, when I think of that whole pregnancy, it seems as far away as early childhood. I remember that night. And I remember how, two weeks later, my morning temp was 98+, which is one-tenth of a degree too low, and I thought, "Well, maybe it's just as well. Jeff is sick, and we've been fighting lately about moving. Maybe it's just as well to wait a month or two, when it's all settled." But the morning after that my temp was above 98.3, and I thought, "Like f— it was just as well!" And I remember worrying about telling my mother, and some of my friends, because I wasn't stopping at two, and I remember the load that dropped when my mother gave her blessing. And that April day coming back from the doctor's; I lay on the bench outside, put my hand on my belly, looked up at the sun and, for the first time, fully let in the happiness. And then, sitting out on the grass with the neighbors, getting into the spirit. Happy. That's how I feel when I'm preg. Happy, always happy. Even when I'm sad, I'm happy. Meaning, even when I'm *pretending* to be sad, or mad, I'm really happy. I just hope I get the chance to be preg again. I just hope.

This is ridiculous, I sometimes try to tell myself. Why not just live my life and forget about getting preg until it happens?

Why not "be here now"? Why not just live my life.

The answer is simple: because I don't *like* my life right now. Because my life right now has no baby-ness in it. I shouldn't have to just live a life with no baby-ness in it when I just pushed out a baby. So: if I can't have baby, baby, and if I can't be preg, then at least I want to be *trying* to be preg.

March 19, 1978

Today all the symptoms are coinciding. Basal temp the lowest of the low, 97⁺, Tes-Tape a dark green forest. The last symptom is subsiding as of two hours ago so I think what happened was I ov'd early this morning. The next few days will tell. Jeff still insists on waiting an extra month, so it doesn't matter if I missed the ov. The thing is: I can get preg (or try to) in 4 to 6 weeks.

Scared, as usual, that something will happen to Jeff before the next ov. Not as terrified as before, but still scared. And scared that something will happen to him before the next baby's *born*. Just got to give me and my family at least one more healthy baby. Just got to.

Sometimes I feel as though I'm *supposed* to be intellectual, or political, or interesting, but I don't *want* to be intellectual, political, or interesting. All I want is my baby. After I get my baby, then I can be intellectual, political, and interesting again. With a baby to dip my hands into, with real live red screaming baby, I can be as intellectual, political, or interesting as they want.

Just got to keep my world together until I can give it baby, baby. Just gotta give Jeff, Elle, and my mother at least one more baby, baby. Just gotta.

March 20, 1978

The symptoms continue to be what they're s'pozed to be. Morning temp up to 97.6$^+$, Tes-Tape paling, Cerv less accessible, sitting back like an ol' granny in the rocker, resting from its work.

We hope. We hope. As I said to Jeff last night, if it weren't for my history of God pulling switcheroo's on me, I'd say I definitely ov'd. Cur-razy.

I also have fears of missing the *next* ov. And other fears. Especially thinking that, a year ago, we were going through the same thing.

But I push onward, anyway. I continue. It's not that I'm a strong woman. It's not that I'm great, or to be admired. *All* women in my position are like this. You should see them at the UNITE meetings. Such is the desire of so many women for children. It's not unique, it's not creative, it's just strong. So strong.

How can I convey to those who don't know what it is? To want to be preg, to give birth, to have a baby? No matter that I already have two healthy children. No matter at all. No matter if I had ten. I want baby, baby, as I wanted baby, baby ten years ago. How can I convey this?

And how can I convey how glad, how relieved, I am to be fertile again? To have my power back?

They say there's no such thing as perfect happiness, that there's only the *anticipation* of happiness. Not so, I say. Baby, baby is perfect happiness.

I guess I could say that baby, baby, and oving, means to me what menstruation means to some feminists.

I feel closer to the next baby now. In one month. We hope; we hope. Then I'll breathe easy, sit back and relax, plunge forward and arrange poetry readings, go thrift shopping, distribute my book, and mourn Kerin properly. Then I'll have my mind back. In one month. I just had a baby and I'm going to have a baby. We hope. We hope.

Take off your undies, and start in with your ovaries!

March 21, 1978

First day of spring. 65°—but it does me no good. For God *did* pull a switcheroo on me. This morning my temperature was 97.3. Back to the ol' drawing board. I don't know how he did it, but he did it. All the symptoms were there. All. And I'm an expert in the business. I know I wasn't imagining things. I know I wasn't exaggerating. Those symptoms were there.

Of course, maybe I really did ov and the *temperature* is wrong. But I know from past experience that can't be. Also, a cold, or other outside factors, wouldn't make the temp *lower*. Okay, maybe I'm getting *closer* to the ov. Maybe. But in that case, so what? Even if I ov tomorrow, it's still three days later than I thought it was. And every day counts. That's something no one, not even my future self, realizes. Every day counts. It *hurts* to not be preg. An empty uterus hurts.

Today for the first time I was in a mood when I just assumed I wasn't ever going to have another baby. I was bitter; all hope was gone. I even thought I could convince myself I no longer cared if I had another baby, so wrung out was I. If I tried really hard, I thought, maybe I could convince myself I no longer wanted a baby. And then maybe I could convince God, too. Then maybe he'd let me ov, and then *I* could pull a switcheroo.

I'm running out of pep talk, out of metaphors, out of poems. I'm tired of hoping, tired of being brave, tired of trying not to worry too much so it won't interfere with my oving, tired of waiting, tired of describing how I feel. I just want a baby. I just want my baby.

I'll never stop loving Kerin. I'll always love her. And I feel so sorry for her I can't stand it. Such a sweet little baby. Such exquisite hands and such a mischevious little face. (Yes, Jeff and I agree, she definitely would have been mischevious.) Such an exquisite baby. I'll never stop feeling sorry for her; I'll never forget the horror.

But I can't do anything about that any more. I wasn't smart enough to save her so I'm certainly not smart enough to bring her back. I can't do anything for her now. All I can do is have another baby. Even if it *was* my fault, I can only make up for it by doing right by my next baby. I can only hope for another chance.

I don't want a job. I don't want a book published. I don't want Guatamalen tops. I just want a baby. I resent anyone who wants me to be intellectual, who wants me to "benefit" from this "experience". I just want a baby. I just want my baby.

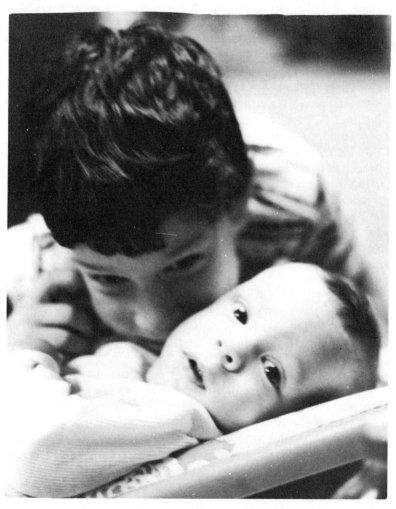

Arin & "L'il Fetus" (Bret)

March 23, 1978

Eileen at the UNITE meeting last night: "I just wish it would all be over, with the baby 'n' all. I just wish it would end. . . I'm nervous, and that's not good for the baby. . . I peeked over at the chart and it said 117. That's normal for a fetal heartbeat, isn't it? . . . I feel nauseous. Oh, I'm sure everything's all right. It's just that . . . No, I can't concentrate on anything. The only people I like to talk to are the people here. And I'm afraid to drive anywhere, 'cause a sudden jerk can cause placenta abrupta. . . Oh, I wish it were over. . . . I know God had his reasons, but I'd like to know what they were. I want some answers. . . I don't know. Maybe it seems silly, but I'd like to prove I can do it. Have my own . . . I can't sleep or anything. . . I just wish it were over. I wish the soap opera would end. . . ."

More than anyone else at UNITE, my heart goes out to Eileen. I'm not sure why. Maybe it's because she's older, and I'd like to have babies after I'm 40. Maybe it's because of her nervousness. Like mine, about getting pregnant again. Last night she turned to me and whispered, "How're ya doing this week?"

"Eh," I shrugged, "thinking about getting pregnant, as usual."

"Oh, I *know*," she said, in a sort-of a motherly way.

"In fact, tonight's the night I'm allowed to!" I added.

'Oh," she laughed. "Are you fertile?"

"No," I answered. "That's the problem. It's just that it's now three months post-partum and that's when the doctors said I could get pregnant again."

During this latter exchange, we clasped hands. It just seemed so natural to reach out. I'm not the type to be physical with people other than Jeff, Elle, and Arin, but there are times when it just seems so natural—to reach out. Like to the nurse when I was in labor with Elle, and Dee during the Dyke-tactics trial, when the jury announced the verdict.

Anyway, maybe I'll get Eileen's 'phone number and call her. I suspect we may have something to give each other.

God's doing it again. The Tes-Tape's getting darker. The temperature is still low. Mucus abundant, sort-of, but not clear.

God's gonna do it again.

Only *this* time, I say, I won't be fooled. This time I'll know. This time I won't expect the temp to stay up.

Oh yeah? says God. You know damn well it *might not* be a false alarm this time.

But this time I'll be cautious, I answer.

You were cautious *last* time, snaps God, and did it help?

As I once said in a poem, I didn't tempt Providence, but Providence was tempted anyway.

Well, I may be fooled, but I'll never let *God* know it. I lie low. Talk little, stay in bed a lot. Lying under the covers is almost like being unconscious. Or non-existent.

The moment I know I'm preg, God will disappear into thin air. Just like, when I was an adolescent, the moment I was asked out on my first date, Fate disappeared. My, we human beings are strong. We grieve easily, we hope easily, but when the grief and the hope are over, we instantly recover.

Dream: *In my mother's house, rain is coming slanted through the back windows. There is as much rain as though we were outside because it is coming horizontal. My sister is laughing and my mother is crying. We all rush to the other side of the house but the rain is coming in there, too, and in exactly the same manner. Besides, a monkey has jumped in the window. It is not exactly a flying monkey, but its rate of descent is slightly less than according to the laws of physics.*

Another dream: *The new house is shiny and modern but it's raining green paint through the windows and staining the furniture. Besides, the house is in the suburbs. Walking around the neighborhood with my mother, I muse, "What'm I gonna do here? What's there for me to do? Oh, next year I'll have a baby, but what'm I gonna do with myself this year?"*

Oh no, not a *school* dream?! At *this* time in my life?! No, I can't cope, I simply can't cope with a school dream *now*. Go to the office and tell them I'm dropping out 'til next September. Tell them I'll go back when I'm preg.

Dream: *To time contractions, use a watch with a second hand. For a stillbirth, use a watch with neither a second hand nor minute hand nor hour hand, and wear it for the rest of your life.*

Dream: *Sound cannot travel in a vacuum. To know what true horror is, go into a vacuum and speak.*

Dream: *If we thrust my dying mother into the third universe before she dies, then she will die in loneliness. But if we let her die in our arms, then she will die in terror, knowing where we will thrust her after she dies. In fact, if we thrust her there at all, we will be in terror forever after, for her body will keep passing above us in the sky, like the moon or a constellation.*

Dream: *A woman I'm visiting has a 4-year-old daughter, a baby, and several crib deaths behind her. I keep noticing that the baby stops breathing for short periods. At one point, it cries and she prepares to feed it. Suddenly it stops crying, and breathing, and the woman tells me wearily, "Oh, it'll probably die before I get its food ready."*
"Aren't you breast-feeding?" I ask.
"No, I never breast-feed any more," she answers. "Then I get too attached and it hurts me even more when they die."

Dream: *I am about to start pushing. It's in my old bed at my mother's house and the furniture is arranged the way it was that year I was about ten and decided (*this was in real life*) to stand at the foot of the bed and fall forward and catch myself by pushing my hands against the nearby wall. And I missed the wall and fell to the floor and lost my breath for a minute or two. Anyway, I am about to start pushing and somebody says, "Hey, I know an easy way to do it!" And she shows me. I lie on my stomach and sort-of roll on it in a certain way. The baby shoots out painlessly in one second: cord, placenta, and all. I rush to pick it up from the floor, in the same spot where I fell as a kid. There it is, my little boy post-mature baby, with "diminished vernix," "an abundance of scalp hair,' clear skin* *and big eyes. It isn't breathing. But I'm not worried. Like with Elle. I try to suck the mucus out of its nose. Something comes out but it still doesn't breathe. "Hey, somebody!" I scream. "Help me out!" Deep down inside I know everything will be all right. Like with Kerin.*

April 2, 1978

So here it is, April—the month I've been waiting for, the month I hoped would be baby-month. But of course that's impossible. For even if I ov tomorrow, and even if I have a 28-day cycle this time, baby-day will still be May 1.

There is, however, some ray of hope. Yesterday Jeff and I did some more doctor-interviewing and we found one who seems to be really careful. He examined me and said I should be oving within the week. He even examined the mucus under a microscope.

So *now* I'm afraid God'll pull *another* switcheroo. But at least it'll look more suspicious now. I mean, God wouldn't pull a switcheroo on a *doctor*, would he?!

I keep saying I can't take much more. But I know that's not true. I can take it; I just don't *want* to. I can take it. There's no end to how much "the human spirit" can take. God *makes* it like that. This way he can dish out as much as he pleases, for our "human spirits" to take.

I'm so tired of being not happy. It's not being sad I mind so much; it's the being not happy. I miss being happy.

And I want to burst forth. I want to go thrift shopping for baby clothes and I want to do spring cleaning and I want to arrange poetry readings. I want to burst forth. I want to get preg so I can be happy so I can burst forth. There's one disadvantage when you "know thyself", when you know what you want. One disadvantage—and that's: There's nothing to be done when you can't *get* what you want. I can't convince myself that when I want is meaningless because it isn't. When I was having PhD troubles, and publishing troubles, I could do that, but not with this.

Four months ago I was anxiously and happily awaiting contractions. Now I'm waiting to *ov*. It all seems so hopeless. I'm so tired.

It's like I always knew it was coming. And yet I didn't. I was *less* worried during any of my pregnancies than most women. I definitely *didn't* know it was coming. But sometimes when I remember back, it *seems* as though I did. I super-impose what I now know upon my pregnancy memories. That's what's so frustrating. It's as though I knew all along—as I was going for pre-natal appointments, as I was shopping for baby-things, as I was lying on my side hugging my big belly—it's as though I knew all along, but wasn't doing anything about it.

April 3, 1978

Depressed today. Reality is stagnant. Afraid God's going to pull another switcheroo. Reality is stagnant. Four months ago I gave a reading at McGlinchey's. I ran into Gil, who said, "I hear you're about to have another child. And I hear you're having trouble."

"Oh no!" I laughed. "I'm not having any trouble. That was just the morning sickness, a long time ago. No trouble at all. I'm fine."

Reality is stagnant. No baby—inside or out. No Kerin. No bassinette next to our bed. No excitement. No warmth. Much ado about nothing. Reality is stagnant. No matter when I ov, I have to wait 'til the next ov. Is this discouragement keeping me from oving?

Reality is stagnant? Is it a premonition, or just a fear? That God plans to kill Jeff the night before baby-night. That this new doctor will want to do test after test on me, until I really *am* too old to have a baby. And Jeff will agree. "We have to be careful," he'll say. "I don't want it to happen again." The doctor will nod. And I'll be able to do nothing but watch as these two men plan the fate of my body. Reality is stagnant. I don't even have Kerin to comfort me. Reality is stagnant.

Friendship is like china
Costly, rich, and rare.

Once broken it can be mended.
But the crack is still there.

Yes, true, the crack is still there, but we can, not patch it, but cover it. Cover it with something pretty. Reality is stagnant. I wasn't meant to bear children, said Anais Nin. I wasn't meant to be a lover of children; I was meant to be a lover of men—oh! shit! I say. I don't want anyone deciding what I *was meant* to do. I'm not meant to do anything; it's what I *mean* to do. Reality is stagnant. What percentage of women who have children lose one of them? I mean a baby, at birth? What percentage, I demand. How much of a coincidence *is* it? How suspicious *is* the whole business? Reality is stagnant. The doctor said I would ovulate within the week. But I just know God's gonna pull another switcheroo. Deep down inside, I know he won't, he can't, but then again, maybe he will. Reality is stagnant. I'm scared. I feel as though I'm tied up. I'm tied up and someone is dangling a knife over my head and saying, "Don't worry; I won't drop it." I'm scared. Reality is stagnant. I'm scared.

Lazarus, I dare you
to look upon my face.

April 4, 1978

Persistent Spinnbarkeit. *That* didn't happen before. So this isn't a tease, right? This is the real McCoy.

It's only recently, I keep telling myself. It's only recently my life has been a nightmare. It's only the past 101 days. It's not my whole life, just the *last* part. Just the past 3½ months. Not my whole life.

April 5, 1978

Everything points to it. And I mean everything. And the more everything points to it, the more I fear the switcheroo.

Still, it remains true that yesterday—as I was shopping with the kids in Children's Outlet, as I stook looking at the Health-Tex shirts in Arin's size—yesterday, unless God pulls a switcheroo, yesterday, around 4:00 p.m., I ov'd.

I actually felt it. I'm convinced. I felt that egg come out. It wasn't Mittelschmerz; it wasn't sharp pains, it wasn't pains at all. And it wasn't over a period of several hours, it was all concentrated in those few minutes. I felt, well, it was sort-of like gas pains and sort-of like muscle pains and sort-of like the cervix opening up and sort-of like contractions. And then suddenly I grew hot, and then, I'm convinced, I felt that egg come out. On the right side. Really.

And then everything quickly but gradually subsided, and I felt as though my body had worked hard. Not me, just my body. I also felt like I do when I've had an orgasm. Finished. Satisfied.

I wasn't imagining. I felt the egg burst through.

Just to make sure, though, when I got home, around two hours later, I did the Tes-Tape bit, and yes, it came out dark, darker than two weeks ago, even. It didn't take five minutes for the dark to run all over the tape; I watched it happen before my very eyes. It hasn't been that dark since the day Arin was conceived.

Still, all last night and when I first got up this morning, I was scared of the switcheroo. It's happened before, I thought. God's done it before. All that has to happen, I thought, was I could take my temp and it could be 97.3. Again. That's all. No explanation. No explanation given, no explanation required.

But the temp was 97.9⁻, which indicates a gradual rise. (Yesterday it was 97.6.) So it's good. Good.

So far. For tomorrow that temp has got to be above 98. And I betcha, I just betcha, it isn't. I mean, why *should* it be? I mean, it should be, but suppose it isn't? Just suppose it isn't?

I take nothing for granted any more. The only reason I'm confident the sun will rise tomorrow morning is that I don't *care* if the sun rises tomorrow morning.

Still: one big, beautiful ov. As beautiful as an orgasm. As beautiful as a labor contraction. One, big, enormous, scrumptous, fantabulous, beautiful ov. All mine.

April 6, 1978

No switcheroo this time (at least not yet). 98$^+$ this morning. And everything else is falling into place. Spinnbarkeit all dried up. Tes-Tape takes an hour to turn green. No switcheroo this time, right? I won't wake up to 97.3 or 97.6 tomorrow, will I?

I actually feel sort-of-happy. I'm not preg but I did ov. (Two more high-temps will tell for sure.) I'm not preg, but I'm also not sterile. And next month, next month, I'll be preg. Right?

To celebrate, I'm buying a "little unda-shirt" in Children's Outlet—they have them on sale. And Jeff and I are going out for dinner. And I'm calling up Drexel and asking about teaching that Advanced Engineering Math course next year. Just as soon as that temp has been high for three days.

No switcheroo this time. Right? Right?

Dee's lesbian-custody trial comes up tomorrow, and Jeff and I are testifying. We're sort-of-character witnesses. I'm glad for this opportunity to do something for the women's movement, as I don't have much else to give it at this time.

April 9, 1978

98.2, 98.1, and 98.5$^+$. Definitely no switcheroo. That was an ov, all right.

But I discovered the chapter in Williams on hypertension in pregnancy. Even by itself, without any other signs of pre-eclampsia or eclampsia, it means something. And, they seem to think, it always indicates some degree of placental insufficiency. B— supposedly goes by Williams but I guess they goofed in my case. Surely they must have goofed in other people's cases, too. Surely it wasn't just that they didn't like *me*.

So B— killed my baby. B—, the feminist, family-centered place to have a baby, killed mine. That makes it even harder to bear. Everytime my blood pressure went up I asked them, I *asked* them, "Is that okay?" and they said, "Oh, yes, nothing to worry about." They always assume everything's okay. They're so enamored with natural family-centered birth that they kill the babies. They killed my baby.

Jeff and I have already written two letters, trying to make them change. Now we'll write a third one, about that chapter in Williams. A whole chapter on hypertension. We don't want to sue; we want them to change.

They killed my baby, and they've possibly ruined me. "A baby is not a gut," I once wrote in a poem. But maybe it is. Maybe it is. Even ten years from now, will a day ever go by that I don't think about it? What about an hour?

And will I be able to have another baby? This time the placenta started to age around the 38th, 39th week. This time they could easily have saved her. But suppose that was the last time they could have saved the baby. Suppose the rest of the times the placenta goes much earlier. Suppose I have to have an actual premature baby next time. I just assume it'll die. I just assume that now.

When Arin was about a month old, I had this nightmare. In it I heard Arin crying and I couldn't find him. Finally I located him in an old locker. *"And as I woke up,"* I wrote in my diary the next morning, *"with dreadful thoughts of what might have been, the most dreadful thought of all was that Arin, among other things, was an object and, like any other object, he could get lost."*

I am an object. Jeff is an object. The egg, sperm, uterus, and ovaries are objects. I'm scared. Will one of these objects get lost? I'm scared.

Dee won her case. She got her 12-year-old baby back. I doubt it was my testimony that made the difference but it was fun testifying. They asked how many children I had and I mentioned Kerin. Meanwhile I got to see some of the dykes again. Dian, the lesbian separatist, had tears in her eyes as we talked about my baby. Seems her little brother died when he was six months old.

I didn't get to discuss the case, in private, with Dee yet. She just right away took Kippy off to celebrate. I also didn't get to tell her about the ov. I want to call her today. Maybe, to celebrate both events, we'll go thrift shopping.

L'il Fetus, tiny tiny object, somehow I'll find you.

April 10, 1978

At night, just as I'm about to drop off to sleep, wanting a baby and getting a baby seem to be one and the same thing.

April 11, 1978

I always had a feeling I wouldn't fit in even with B—. It's true. I always had this feeling I'd be the only feminist who didn't fit in with B—. Someday, I felt, I'd have a fight with them or something. Why can't I have one thing, just one thing, in my life that's just plain happiness? Why must everything be different, something to write about?

B— killed my baby. I'm 5 days late, the head is engaged, my blood pressure is steadily rising, and Dr. N— tells me to make an appointment for "after Christmas". More than one week from then. Knowing what I know now, having read two obstetrics texts, it really does seem as though he were purposely trying to kill my baby. He couldn't have been, but it really does seem that way.

And also, could that rejection letter the day before have

had anything to do with it? It says in Williams, "ambulation has no place in the treatment for hypertension in pregnancy." Could my excitement have constricted the placental blood vessels even more? Did my being a writer kill my baby? Is everything I do destined to make my life even worse? Is everything I do doomed? Is God playing with me?

The closer I get to the next pregnancy, it seems, the harder reality sinks in. Is this because, when I get preg again, it'll sort-of be as though I'm giving up on Kerin coming alive again?

B— killed my baby. I'm not just saying that to alleviate any guilt feelings *I* might have. B— *did* kill my baby. Now Kerin won't get to do anything. Her clothes, Elle's hugs, Arin's rambunctiousness, my milk—it'll all go to another baby. She wanted to be our baby so badly; I just sense it. She knew what was waiting for her, and she tried so hard to get to it. And B— killed her.

It seems as though it's been forever. Not that time is passing slowly, but that I can't imagine anything *else*. It seems like forever, but then so did my childhood, my virginity, the times when I was trying to conceive, my pregnancies. It seems like forever but, I tell myself, so did a lot of things (*e.g.*, Camp, when I was a kid. It was an endurance test.) It seems like forever but, I keep telling myself, so did a lot of things. It will end, I say, and then maybe I'll even forget. Even when I read this notebook over, I'll forget. Like I always forget about giving birth. It'll end, I repeat. I'll get preg and have another baby and it'll end. I *will* have another baby. It will end. I will be happy again.

It'll end. It'll end.

April 14, 1978

In four days I get my period. I'm sort-of looking forward to that.

Okay, it's all been said. *The Bereaved Parent*. That's the name of the book. It's all there. Everything I've been writing about. "Grief and Powerlessness," "Grief and Fear," "Grief and the Rest of Your Life." It's all been said.

All, that is, except Grief and the Demons. Yeah, what

about Grief and the Demons? What about the Demons? Huh?
What about the Demons?

And also, food. Grief and food. There does seem to be
some connection between grief and food; I'm not sure what it
is. I just know that, after my father died, I wrote a poem called
"The Kitchen." It was about how Jeff and I went grocery
shopping for my mother, and how all the things on her list
made me feel weepy. I wanted the food to be able to comfort
her, somehow. And the warm yam syrup, crazy as it may seem,
is what brought on the first tears concerning my father's death.
I also know that after my baby died, I said I wasn't interested
in eating. I *could* eat but wasn't interested. And my mother
cooked supper, and later said to me, "Well, you enjoyed the
chicken and broccoli. . ." I don't know. . .the way she said the
word "enjoyed". As though, again, she wanted the food to
somehow comfort me.

Maybe it's just the "Jewish-mother-chicken-soup" syn-
drome. I don't know. But there is definitely a connection between grief and food. Definitely.

April 15, 1978

Something funny happened today. I got my period three
days early. Eleven days after oving, instead of fourteen. I don't
know why. It's never happened before. But it's probably for
the better. It might make the next ov, the baby-ov, happen
three days earlier.

It feels good to feel the blood dripping. It's a real period
this time (not just post-partum bleeding). One real period. One
big scrumptuous bright-red dripping dark-red generous schloshy
beautiful fantabulous supercalifragilisticexpioladocious period.
All mine. I've got my power back. I've got a potential baby.
Now I feel what the dykes are saying when they talk about the
power of woman's blood.

One big scrumptous period, and hopefully, the *last* period
for a long, long time.

April 18, 1978

Dee about my ov: "Oh, fantastic!   Oh Marion, that's just fantastic! That's. . .fantastic!"

Dee, about my period: "Oooo--I'm so excited for you!"

April 20, 1978

I feel so anxious, so afraid. This fear won't prevent me from getting preg, because once I've ov'd, and once we've done all we can do, I'll relax. I just feel nervous waiting.

I've always been a do-er, a get-right-down-to-it-er. Like in school, with exams and term papers. I always started the assignment as soon as I knew about it. I hated cramming, and I hated procrastinating. Both made me nervous.

But *this* is out of my control. If it were up to me, I'd ov right now. I'd keep on oving and keep on trying until I made it. This waiting, this procrastinating, this last-minute cramming has made me unnerved. It's out of my control. And although it won't be my fault if we don't make it this time, I'll *feel*—not as though it *is* my fault, but as though God *thinks* it is my fault. As though God, like a teacher, is saying, "Now, see? You didn't try hard enough this time. So now I want you to spend the next month thinking about how you didn't really try hard enough. Then maybe you'll learn your lesson."

As usual, I feel helpless, powerless, frustrated. In this last lap (we hope!) I'm anxious and afraid. Afraid I'll ov the next time *without* the temp going down, or Tes-Tape turning dark, or Cerv opening. Afraid God will sneak the ov past me. Also afraid Jeff will be inaccessible when I ov. Afraid God *sees* that baby-day is approaching and has something planned. Like an accident.   Or one of us getting arrested (they'll let him go the next day, but so what?).

Thoughts like these are with *all* of us, deep deep down. But right now I feel them at the surface. At the surface, and strongly. How can I convey it? How can I convey?

It occurs to me that this is the third time I'm anxious about conceiving (I wasn't anxious when trying to conceive Kerin) but the first time I'm keeping a journal about it. My first trying-to-conceive journal. I guess I was destined to keep a trying-to-conceive journal.

I had fun announcing my ov at the UNITE meeting. We went around the room, as usual, each of us telling what had happened in the past two weeks. So I said, "I don't know whether I should say this in mixed company, but last week I— shall we say?—regained my fertility!" Some of the women clapped!

April 22, 1978

I think about two lines from two poems I wrote last year, after my father died. One was "Will I dream that the next child I carry becomes my father?" The other was "What heirloom will I inherit for my 35th birthday?" It all turns my blood cold.

We're over Jeff's parents house for the first time since my life was divided in half. It feels different. Depressing. Nothing interests me. I can't concentrate on anything. Will I ever be happy again? Just as long as I didn't miss my ov, I'm willing to give it a try.

Now I understand why people get drunk. Now I understand.

April 23, 1978

I don't jitter, but I feel jittery. As though I'm waiting in line. Worrying doesn't help, people would say. But somehow I feel that it might.

I feel as resentful and envious of women with three children as a childless woman might feel of women with *one* child. And I would prefer to be unconscious. And when I can't be unconscious, I would prefer to be still.

In this last lap, I find myself more nervous than ever. I think backwards a lot, think about Kerin a lot. All they had to do was induce labor in the 39th or 40th week. Murderers! In this last of the last lap, I miss my little baby. She'd be four months old. Probably just starting to fit into a Carter's medium. Turning over and starting to grow up. It makes me sad to think that, even if the hospital were to call up and tell us it was all a mistake, it was some other baby that died, it makes me sad to think that Kerin would now be four months old. And, among other things, it would be very difficult for me to start nursing her.

In this last of the last lap, I find life hard to live. BUT: I'm glad it *is* the last of the last lap. I'm glad it isn't December anymore, or January. I'm glad I'm closer to the next baby. Because of *course* there really isn't anything to be nervous about; it's just that I *feel* nervous. Of *course* this is fear I'm feeling, not a premonition. Of course I'm getting closer to the next baby. Right? We're closer to the next baby, right? Right?

April 25, 1978

So? should I now go around writing poems and articles about how B— killed my baby and about the significance of blood pressure in pregnancy? Should I get political? I don't feel like it; don't really feel like it. I'm not in the mood. Maybe when I'm preg. But then again, maybe not.

B— killed my baby. I don't want to live. Living means pretending to be happy. Or, worse yet, actually *being* happy. Living means forgetting. Living means fooling myself. And I'm too well-adjusted for that.

And I feel downright insulted. B— didn't think enough of me to be careful with my baby. They raped me, used my body as an instrument of death. Used my body as a weapon to suffocate my baby.

When I walk the streets, if perchance I feel hopeful and smile, then I imagine that God is saying to me, in a mocking tone, "How can you be so happy when I just killed your baby?" To live is to kid myself. B— killed my baby, pure and simple. That will always be true.

So what do I do now? Devote my life to spreading the gospel about the significance of rising blood pressure in pregnancy? Have my life be determined, not by myself, but by my circumstances? I always believed that was politically wrong, and I still do. I mean, rising blood pressure in pregnancy is important, but it's no more important than curing cancer, or the abolition of capital punishment, or the Politics of Motherhood, or any of the other causes. I never did approve of isolating causes. Like charities. Like the Kennedy's supporting research about retarded children because they have a retarded sister. Like the mothers of retarded children volunteering their services to the Retarded Children's Organization, becoming president and all that. It's all so subjective, so nationalistic. All the charities just wind up competing against each other for donations, media coverage, etc. What they should do is unite and fight for social change, *all* social change. Of course I want Kerin's Death To Have Some Meaning, but I want it to have the *right* meaning.

So what do I do now? Yes, I know it's April 25, and Day 14 is approaching, but B— still killed my baby. And I'm still afraid God's planning to sneak the ov past me. That mucus is very definitely scant and thick and non-Spinnbarkeit-y and the temp very definitely has not dropped and the Tes-Tape is very definitely not a dark bluish-green. But I *could* still wake up tomorrow, and the next day and the next, to temps over 98. No explanation required. It could just happen. I don't trust anything. And the only reason God lets the sun rise every morning, the only reason he doesn't snitch it from us during the night, is he knows the people in China are there to check it, to keep track of it.

I just keep on writing. I don't suffer while I'm writing. I don't feel nervous. I don't feel what I'm writing *while* I'm writing. Like when I go to UNITE meetings. Or talk about it to *anybody*. I just keep on writing, and reading what I write, and not believing it.

April 26, 1978

Arin's been acting up. Going through a bad stage. The "terrible four's". It was the same with Elle. Only with Elle, I also had a baby in the house.

He's just too big. They're both too big. I didn't feel that way before. I thought each age had its own special charm. "Kids're just so *funny*," I'd lingo. Now I feel they're just too big, too mischevious, too elusive.

I try not to unconsciously hold them back, keep them babies. I try to let them know of my feelings, without getting us all obsessed with them. "Arin, you *haf*ta keep lettin' me hava cheek until we have the next baby," I laugh, and "Elle, you just hafta bea kid one more year. Then you can get too big for your britches if you want." I try to keep everything honest and healthy, without going overboard. But I guess that's a contradiction. In order to be honest, I *have* to go overboard.

Every part of me wants a baby. Every thought I have is just one more reason I want a baby. And they're all *healthy* reasons. I wish they could be *un*healthy reasons so I could talk myself out of them.

"But didn't you sign something when you first went to B— saying you agreed to do everything naturally?" two people have been stupid enough to ask. In answering them, I wouldn't know where to begin. (1) "No, we didn't sign anything; they gave us nothing to sign and if they had we wouldn't have gone there." (2) " 'Natural' means no pain-killing drugs given without permission, and that's all." (3) "Natural doesn't mean no pre-natal care. If it did, they wouldn't have pre-natal appointments.' (4) "B— has plenty of unnatural things: *e.g.*, they induce labor, they do C-sections, they monitor, they use epidurals and Demerol, and, when I had Arin, they tried to get me to take Nembuthol—were quite pushy about it, in fact—said I was having false labor because I was 3 cm. Well, *everyone* in early labor is three centimenters! I refused the Nembutol, and had Arin within six hours. This exact same thing happened with at least two other mothers that very same evening." (5) "If we wanted everything natural, we would have had a home birth."

Mainly, though, the question makes me wonder whether there are people at B—, infiltrators, who—like FBI agents who join organizations they consider subversive—are trying to perpetuate the myth that natural means dangerous. In other words, I'm wondering—now, I know this sounds crazy--I'm wondering whether they purposely kill babies and then say, or allow others to say, "But you wanted it natural. . ." I don't really *want* Kerin to be a political victim but I wonder if she is.

Stories. People tell me stories. Against their better judge-
ment, probably, but I understand how they can't resist it. The
one Freda told me the other night was the last straw. Pregnancy
for me will never be the same. A friend of hers was five months
preg with her third, and one evening, while visiting Freda, she
felt the baby kick violently for a few minutes and then stop
moving altogether. When a few days went by and the baby still
hadn't moved, she went to the doctor, and yes, the baby had
died. It would be too dangerous to take it in the fifth month,
the doctor said; she'd have to wait 'til she aborted spontaneous-
ly. (Ya know, people on the streets seeing her big belly and
saying, "Congratulations." Ya know.) So for two more months
she carried that dead baby. But, assured the doctor, the whole
thing was just a fluke. Probably a cord accident. So she got
pregnant again, and, yes, it happened again. Exactly the same
thing. Horrible. Horrible. But she decided to try again—and,
yes, it happened yet again. Talk about Kafkaesque. The
world's best obstetricians were stymied. Each time she carried
around a dead baby for two months. Unlike me, she *does* have
something to lose by trying again. Which she probably will, in a
few years. Maybe her body will be different then, she hopes.
After all, she did have two healthy children, two uncomplicated
pregnancies and births. Maybe, she hopes. If I have any idea,
Freda tells me, any at all, please let her know. Please.

So now I know, once and for all, that pregnancy and birth
are not accomplishments, but privileges. Like money. Like
prestige. Like power. It's something that a woman is *given*. It's
not something to be proud of. It's not *up* to us. Yes, the next
pregnancy will be different for me. Not only because I'll be
fearful—I may *not* be—but because I now know too many
things.

BUT: not only is it April 28, but my temp's been low for
two days in a row. The ov—the ov—is imminent.

April 29, 1978

I wish, I wish, I would *suddenly* ov, like last time. I wish, I wish, I'd feel the egg come out.

Listen. Feel. Pay attention to your body. Like a heartbeat. I can hear it if I listen. Sssh. Ssssh.

May 1, 1978

I think I caught the egg before it dropped. I think I ov'd and I think I'm preg. At any rate, I think I ov'd.

May 2, 1978

Baby. Oh baby, baby. Are you in there, sweetheart?

May 3, 1978

Yes, I might be preg. And it's a good feeling, to might-be-preg. In spite of myself I catch myself being happy. And, as usual during the post-ovulatory phase when I'm trying to get preg, I catch myself with my hand on my stomach. "It's too soon for that," says Jeff. But my hand goes there, anyway. Because, after all, L'il Fetus might be in there. I have to put some love in there, just in case. Yes, of course I know L'il Fetus would just be a bunch of multiplying cells at this stage, but maybe love gets stored. I have to put some love on the present layer of cells before it gets covered by the next layer.

I've already decided. I *will* go thrift-shopping for baby clothes (as I do now). But I won't baby-shop in regular stores until the baby's actually here, and I won't sew anything. But of course I will allow myself to love and get excited about the baby. How could I not? I could only pretend not to. And, of course, for the very reason that L'il Fetus, like all fetuses, might not live long enough to be my baby. . . well, that's even *more* reason to give it love while it's a fetus.

Maybe I'm not preg. Maybe Jeff's sperm count went down or something. Maybe, after having three babies, my uterus is shaped differently. Dr. F— said it's twice as large as the typical uterus, but that's not uncommon for a multipara. Still, maybe that larger uterus makes it harder to conceive. The sperm has more room to bounce around in before it can get up the Fallopian tubes. Or something. Maybe I'm not preg.

Talk about family planning! I think they're just using women for population control. Because they tell us all about how to *prevent* conception but nothing about how to *produce* it. Then, when we decide we want to get preg, we wait and suffer and get all nervous and, possibly, make matters worse. They tell us all about diaphragms, pills, and IUD's, but they don't tell us that the man's sperm count goes down if he comes too often. So the anxious couple does it every day for a year and nothing happens. So they go to a fertility clinic and *then* are told the big secret, or else they go complaining to friends and relatives, who tell them, "Just relax and you'll get pregnant", and, "Don't *try* to get pregnant and you'll get pregnant." So they "relax"—*i.e.*, they stop doing it every day—and, lo and behold, they get preg. Neither the establishment, nor the women's movement, seems to care much about women having knowledge and control of their own bodies in *that* way. In fact, to get hints on how to conceive, I've had to read books on how *not* to conceive and then do the opposite!

And the suffering of women trying to conceive is not made quite as public as that of women suffering from unwanted pregnancies. Women are not warned of the intensity of the trying-to-conceive suffering; instead, they are urged to wait until they are "really sure"'they want to have a child—so sure that they go crazy trying to have that child. And only then do the fears come crashing in. Only then do they realize that the opposite of contraception is not necessarily conception.

I'm not saying every woman should do what I do, with the temp charts and Tes-Tape. It's just that, when a woman is planning a family and is concerned about whether or not she can have children, and she asks her doctor about it, the doctor almost invariably shrugs his shoulders and tosses her off with "You never know 'til you try." Most of the time *he* doesn't know. And no doctor I know of has ever *offered* any woman advice on how to conceive, although they all jump in with "What type of birth control are you using?"

Gee, I remember when Jeff and I finally decided to have Elle, and I was looking at one of the Margaret Sanger pamphlets and I read "Fertility Clinic: For Couples Planning A Family". Well, *I* thought that meant they gave you little tips on how to conceive, and then examined you to see if you could have babies, and if your body could take a pregnancy, and all that. So I called them up and they asked me, "How long have you been trying?"

"Huh?" I answered. "I haven't been trying at all."

Fertility clinics are only for women who are *already* out of their minds. Just like high-risk obstetricians are only for women who have already experienced tragedy. The very opposite of preventive medicine. Very political.

Getting back to the population control business, I'm not only talking about the woman who has many children, or even more than two children. Our woman might very well be trying for her first pregnancy. Is it population control women are being sacrificed for, or population elimination?!

I just talked to my friend Judy, who's the editor of *Hera*, which is a Philadelphia based feminist newspaper. She wants me to write up this Kerin-business.

I feel dazzled. What should I emphasize? Should I mention B— by name? If so, how do I put it, to avoid getting sued? Should I mail them the letters we wrote to Dr. F— ? Which of my feelings are feminist? The whole project seems so exciting; I think I'll get to work on it right away.

Frustration-dream again. Did L'il Fetus fail to implant? Did it keep bumping into the three implantation sites? Especially Kerin's. Is L'il Fetus afraid to implant? Worse yet, did it implant low?

May 14, 1978

Just a short Mother's Day note.

(1) This is day 2—*i.e.*, I got my period yesterday morning.

(2) We talked to Dr. F— yesterday, and listen to what happened:

After he had us sitting down on the side of the desk on which he wanted us, and we knew he had the B— records in his hands and was about to tell us what was in them—well, he up and said to us, "You know, the whole episode was completely unnecessary—on *everybody's* part." He paused significantly, and my blood and bones froze. I knew he meant *our* part, too.

"Go on," I said.

"Well," he said, staring at the records, "it says here 'Patient was told to come in immediately'..."

"What!" we exclaimed. "We were *not* told to come in immediately."

And so on and so on. They lied on other counts, too. To make them less guilty, and *me more* guilty—*i.e.* it is written in the records that *I* killed my baby.

Dr. F— did believe us. Told us, in fact, that he's a member of a committee which is investigating B—. And, as we left, said to us, "I'm sorry. I'm really sorry." and "I hope you're pregnant."

More on all this later. Right now I've got to work on somehow acting halfway normal, for the sake of my children, husband, and mother-in-law.

May 15, 1978

Funny, I expect to make it the *next* time, and I keep thinking, "How can I possibly wait eleven more days?" When, in fact, it could be many more months, or years, or forever.

Dream: Yes, you have to put it out of your mind, or stop concentrating on it, or *something*.

Summary: B— killed my baby, and is accusing *me* of killing my baby. Plus three days ago I got my period. Okay, now put that out of your mind.

7:00 a.m. One more half-hour to stay in bed. But you can't spend it thinking about *that*. Something else, *any*thing.

School dreams. Yeah, that's it, school dreams. Gee, I have that paper due tomorrow; how *ever* will I get it done? Especially when I don't even know what topic it's supposed to be on.

And gee, I haven't read a book or a newspaper in *such* a long time. Yes, Ma, you were right. It just doesn't feel right, not to have read a book or newspaper in such a long time. I'm not sure *why* it doesn't feel right, but it doesn't; it just doesn't.

Okay, let me have a look in Kerin's crib for a book or a newspaper. Check under the mattress, between the bars. . . .

NO! Can't let that ruin your life. Something else, *any*-thing. . . Gee, working in a day care center sure is hard work. I really want to quit—I want to enjoy this pregnancy—but I have to give two weeks' notice. So many children, so many rooms... and the rooms are so *wooden*, and the windows keep opening... What happened to all the children? Omigod! shut the windows! No, *I* didn't open them; they just keep opening by themselves, and the room gets emptier and emptier, and there are fewer and fewer children. No, *I'm* not losing them; they just keep getting lost by themselves. That's how this day care center works. . .

No, I can't let it ruin my life—*What* life? This feels more like death.

To continue what I was writing about before, B— lied on at least 3 counts:

(1) They said that, when I first called and reported the meconium discharge, they had told me to rush right in, and that I hadn t. And they said I got there at 4:30, whereas I got there at 4:00. There are of course, several things to say about that:

> (a) We have subsequently learned that B—'s procedure for emergencies is to tell the patient to rush in to *Jefferson* (their back up), which I *certainly* would have done, especially since we were at the time only a few blocks from Jefferson.

> (b) Dr. M— contradicted herself during my fourweeks' appointment, by telling us that the reason they did *not* tell us to come in right away was that meconium staining is quite common. 30% to 40% of all babies have it, she said. (She made no distinction between staining and discharge—*i.e.* **thick** meconium.)

> (c) Dr. F— said that, even when I did come in, it wasn't too late to save Kerin.

(d) Once I did come in, they did nothing but monitor. And, of course, Dr. M—'s records say nothing about how they called an anesthesiologist and how he didn't show up until after I had delivered.

(e) What would they have done if I had gotten in at 2:00 instead of 4:00?

(2) They said that we at first refused the monitor, and a lengthy discussion ensued. True, we asked questions about the monitor, but the discussion was not lengthy. And if it had been, certainly they had the power to stop it.

(3) They said that they instituted a pitocen drip to speed up labor. As I said elsewhere, they never actually used pitocen; they "put in an open line" for it, but said they felt I was coming along fast enough. This point, as well as Point 2, could easily be proven, as we have the whole thing on tape.

Now, any woman who has given birth feels that she did a great job, and was very special. She does *not* expect to be accused of killing her baby, especially not on paper or in the courtroom. And she does *not* expect the people present at the birth to be the ones who do the accusing. She does not expect to be accused of not laboring well.

But does all this invalidate the birth experience for me? Does it invalidate *all* my birth experiences? No.

For the *doctor* doesn't make the birth experience; it's the woman and the baby. Also, as I keep saying, childbirth is *rough* beauty. Like all beauty. And any set of facts doesn't average out to *one* fact. You have to just keep the whole set of facts. You can't simplify. That's why I keep writing, all kinds of things, at length. You need it all. It doesn't average out.

Along those lines, here's a conversation Jeff and I had a month or so ago:

Jeff: She was born, she suffered, she died—just like the rest of mankind. (At this, he suddenly looks surprised at himself, to be coming up with that kinda thing.)

Me (laughing): You've *got* to be kidding. (Jeff starts laughing.) Where'dja dig *that* one up?

Jeff: Well, actually, I got that from this fable I once heard. This king or somebody wants to know the history of mankind, and the wise man writes a 30-volume account. When he goes back and shows it to the king, the king says, "Can't you make it a little shorter?" So the wise man shortens it to *one* volume, and shows *that* to the king. But the king still says, "Can't you make it a little shorter?" So the wise man goes and writes on a slip of paper, "He was born, he suffered, he died."

Me: Which is a lot o' crap. Now, if *I* were asked to write a history of *my* life, I would write—

Jeff: You were born, you had a great time, you died.

Me: Nope! I'd write, "I was born, I was interested in math, I fell in love, I pushed out eight babies, one of them died, I—NO, wait a minute! I left out the part about the PhD. And I *haf*ta tell ya about the Walking Method. Plus the Politics of Motherhood—Oh, I'll need one volume, at least—Oh no, wait a sec! What about all my poems?! And you've just gotta hear about Elle, my first. See, we got t' the hospital and I was only two centimeters dilated so they left me in this room, saying something like 'See ya tomorrow morning'—It was my first, see—but then two hours later I rang for the nurse and started in with "Oh. . .oh. . .I hafta go to the bathroom. . .whoa boy, do I hafta go to the bathroom. . .oooh. . ."

Jeff (laughing): Okay, Mar, I get the idea!

May 16, 1978

"Don't make love just to have a baby," some people say. "Why the f— not?!" I counter.

(1) I can *so* enjoy making love at the same time that I'm trying to make a baby. I always did, and I do now. For one thing, the conditions under which it's easiest to make a baby are also the most enjoyable.

(2) It's just a myth that being scientific is inconsistent with enjoyable love-making. So what if the baking-soda solution drips on the fancy negligee? They say sex is supposed to be fun, anyway. And who needs—and who wears—a fancy negligee? What's so terrible about being scientific? And, no matter what, the orgasm is still there. (Assuming it is!)

(3) Anyway, suppose I didn't enjoy baby-fucking? So what? So I can enjoy it for the *rest* of the cycle. Just not those 4 or 5 fertile days.

Relax, they say, don't think about it. They're always telling me not to think. Relax, they say, and just wait. And God echoes. Please, I beg. Anything, I'll do anything. But please don't make me just relax and do nothing.

But God, it appears, *created* woman to "relax" and do nothing. To wait. Only he "forgot" to make us like it.

"It's a good thing I already have two children," I keep thinking.

But somehow, I feel, *they're* part of the plan. Like, maybe God meant for me to have some other kids first, so I could watch helplessly as I ruin *their* lives, as well as mine. But then, why *two* kids? Why not just one?

May 17, 1978

I feel as though God is mockingly saying, "There, you're postponing your life, your happiness. 'Someday, someday,' you keep saying, 'Someday I'm gonna have a baby.' Time's a-passing, kid. Let's *see* that baby."

I can't explain it. It's as though God's gonna punish *me* for procrastinating, whereas *he's* the one who's procrastinating. And even though I know it isn't completely in my power to get preg, I *feel* as though it is. It's a little like, after I had Elle, logically, I knew it wasn't *my* fault if she cried, but I *felt* as though it was. Responsibility with no power. That's how I described it then. That's how it is now. Is that the lot of all women? responsibility with no power. Only waiting, and "relaxing" can accomplish anything. Only time can accomplish anything. Only time. Month and months of time.

Just relax, they say, or, "wait 'til your body's ready." Do I detect a note of sadism in their voices?

I try not to count the days. But how can I not? How can a *whole* day go by without my thinking 'Day 5'? An hour, maybe. But a day? I don't know. . . A day is just so long, so big, so full.

Why do I keep waiting for this horror to end, daydreaming of its end, feeling as though it's ended *now*, and then realizing with a horrifying jolt that it isn't? Why don't I just realize that my life is different now?

B— killed my baby and is accusing *me* of killing my baby. It's happened before; sometimes the mother actually goes to jail.

I'll never have another baby. The doctors won't *let* me. My life is different now. I'll be writing articles about what happened, and, even though all the characters will be anonymous, the doctors will be afraid to touch me. Or else they *will* take my case and, for revenge, *they*'ll kill the baby. Throw it on the floor right after it's been born. Horror, horror. The doctor's won't let me have another baby. My life is different now. It's political now, totally political. There is no room for personal happiness. B— is bigger than I am. It's a business. Like any business, it will play for blood. Like the Mafia. In order to protect itself, it will put me on trial for killing my baby. I'm not a radical for nothing. I know what I say. Some of it is literal, some is figurative, but it's all true in some way. B— is bigger than I am. I can't win. B— will have the doctors and the courts and the government behind it.

I'm afraid. I *need* doctors for the next baby. I need tests, I need pitocen, I need monitoring. I'm afraid. My personal happiness is over. The system is bigger than I am. It will play for blood.

May 18, 1978

I don't go around crying any more and I don't feel frightened any more and I don't wake up in the morning and just not want to get out of bed. I'm more my **usual** kind of sad, like when things just plain aren't going exactly the way I'd like.

May 19, 1978

Talk about nationalistic! Both Jeff and I have been told, by certain people, that "I can see why *you*'d feel the way you do about B—. But *we* still feel good about it and we'll probably have our next baby there."

If it had happened to someone else rather than us, and if

that someone else had told us about it, we would still feel the same way we do. Of course, we wouldn't concentrate on it as much and feel as miserable, but our opinion would be the same. I would still have the same political second thoughts about midwives and maternity centers (namely, their being a part of the system). And I would not have my next baby at B—.

Do people think we're just reacting emotionally? Do they not believe us? Do they think maybe it was our fault? Or do they just believe it couldn't possibly happen to them?

It *isn't* just us, is it? God didn't specifically choose us, and only us, did he? B— *has* killed other people's babies, too—right? It isn't just us? And if it is just us, it's still not our *fault*? Right?

Why do I always have to be different, left out? In situations where people don't believe me? Where they tell me gently "Well, yes, I can understand how you feel, but naturally *I* don't feel that way because it was you, not me."

But anyway, politically, getting back to what I was saying before, I'm always amazed (I don't know why; I should be used to it by now) when I see people forming opinions according to what's happened to *them*. How ethnocentric, how nationalistic, can you get?

May 23, 1978

I can't move them. I used to think 'way back when I was an adolescent, I used to think I could move them. The publishers, the teachers, the doctors. But I can't. I can't. Dr. M— saw me push out a baby and she saw my poems. And she still wasn't moved. She has to save her career, her reputation. She's part of the system. Of *course* I'm not surprised. And yet I am. As Jeff says, she would stop at nothing. If we decided to sue, she might even kill us.

Although I could be preg in a few days, and although sometimes I allow it to give me a jerk of hope, my *feelings* are of despair. We did all we could possibly do to get me preg *last* month. And we *did* get me preg last *year*. What is the point? Huh? What was the point?

8½ years ago I wrote a doctoral thesis. But a doctoral thesis wasn't what they wanted. What they wanted was for me to write a thesis on one of *their* topics. So the fact that I wrote a thesis so quickly, all by myself, made the whole thing take *longer*, not shorter.

But I'm willing for my *professional* life to suffer because I don't fit in. I'm willing for that. But why does *this* have to happen, *too*? I'll probably wind up rocking the boat too much so that the doctors'll probably kill my next baby, too. And me, too, this time. Because I rock the boat, I won't be allowed to rock the cradle.

No, I just don't believe in the next baby any more. It's five months now. It *is* spring. It's almost summer. I don't, in my heart, believe. I don't *dis*believe, either, but I don't believe. But I don't disbelieve. As I said in my adolescent diary, damn hope!

And yesterday I had a revelation. I was thinking about, and trying to remember, how I felt when I was pushing Kerin out—ya know, trying to push her out as fast as possible even though, as I've said, I wasn't actually worried. It was the same as when I see one of the kids fall down and start to cry. I'm not actually worried, but I watch them extra-carefully for a few minutes, anyway. Why?

Well, I was thinking, it's because of the old saying, "God helps those who help themselves." If I watch the kids carefully, God'll reward me by having them not have a concussion. If I push as hard as I can, God'll reward me by having the baby come out breathing. "God helps those who help themselves."

But then I realized that it's not that, it's not the old saying that I believe, that *everyone* believes. It's the converse. Not "God helps those who help themselves" but "God doesn't help those who don't help themselves." Or: "Ya'd better help yerselves—and as much as possible, not as much as necessary—ya'd better help yerselves, or else." So we watch, and we push, and we help ourselves 'til we bust, because we're afraid of what God'll do to us if we don't.

May 25, 1978

If I missed the ov, it's certainly not my fault. It would just be that God falsified the symptoms. Just like B— falsified the records.

May 29, 1978

It all happens at the same time, according to the books. The egg finishes ripening, the mucus plug comes out, sufficient corpus luteum has accumulated, the egg comes out, the mucus "assumes a character suitable for the transmission of sperm". And more, much more, that I can't pronounce, let alone remember. It all hasta happen at the same time; if any *one* of the things *doesn't* happen, conception is impossible.

And what if one of the things doesn't happen? What if an egg ripens but then *another* egg comes out? Or what if the mucus makes a mistake and gets Spinnbarkeit-y too early or too late?

It's worse when you know what to fear. It's easier to have an undefined fear.

June 1, 1978

Holly at UNITE meeting last night: I want to get pregnant—and yet I don't.

Me: I want to get pregnant—and I do!

Yes, I'm now able to Do Other Things—more than I was two or three months ago. That Math Anxiety Worshop is, once again, going really well. And I get all excited thrift-shopping—and yesterday I bought a real moule pillow for $4—and Arin's especially yummy today, even though he's not a baby, and I arranged to buy us all a second-hand refrigerator through the classifieds. And just today I called up Drexel to see about teaching one of their evening graduate courses, and they said yes—they did have me down for one of them. And, of course, there's that poetry reading next week—my first since B— raped me—and I plan to read only poems written during my pregnancy and afterwards. I announced the reading at last night's UNITE meeting, and they asked me to bring my poems to one of the meetings.

So yes, I'm Doing Other Things, and no, I don't need a baby. So why do I feel as though I do?

I guess it's that I *want* a baby so badly—because I just had one—that it's *like* a need. I know how beautiful baby, baby is, so I want it badly. And a great enough want is actually a need.

June 9, 1978

All's well. I ov'd again and I might be preg again. I feel good. All's well until we hear otherwise. Even God is innocent until proven guilty.

June 10, 1978

We timed it right this time. If I ov'd on the 2nd and I'm preg, it's a boy. Otherwise, a girl. Yes, we did time it right. I mean, as long as we do it three days or less before ov-ing, that's timing it right. But somehow I feel as though it's different with us. I feel as though God *expects* more from us, *i.e.*, unless we do it less than *two* days before I ov, and unless we put the sperm right at the opening and unless I lie on my back so virtually no sperm leaks out—I won't get preg. Other people get preg by simply doing it, but God says, mockingly, to me, "Oh, I know you can do better than that." Like teachers in school: "We know that's not your best." The ol' potential bit, like in my "un-schooling" poems. The more you give, the more they want. Like the bosses.

Still 'n' all, I go around assuming we made it. Not that I'm all ecstatic, just that I'm not miserable. I feel as though I'm waiting for nine or so more days from now, when my waking temp will still be high and I *can* be all ecstatic.

I laugh and act witty with my family. I talk when I don't have to. I giggle, then tell Jeff and the kids, "Let me take advantage of this when I can. I mean, all I hafta do is get my period next Saturday and you'll have your mopey Marion back." Then I giggle again.

June 10, 1978

Oh, I'm probably getting my period.
Aw—c'mon—you know damn well you might not be.
Yep, you know damn well you could be preg. After all, all you hafta do is not get your period for another nine days. That shouldn't be so hard. To hold off for nine days.
See, it has to *happen*. It has to happen. Understand?

i.e. I always feel surprised when anything happens. Surprised when I get preg. Surprised when I have a live baby. Surprised when I have a dead baby. It's all surprising. Everything—not only babies. I guess I *am* a bit of an existentialist, I mean, why not nothing.

It has to happen. A period has to happen. So probably it won't. But pregnancy also has to happen. So probably that won't either. In other words, I feel as though I'm not preg but I'm not gonna get my period. Cur-razy.

My mind leaps ahead. I'm supposed to be nervous about this (possible) pregnancy but I'm afraid I just can't pull that bit off. I feel a little like I felt when I was preg with El; I feel like I'm getting preg for the first time. Maybe even more so. My mind leaps ahead. "Preg," I plan to say to F— on the 'phone. Before I even tell her who's calling. (See, the whole business of "preg" started five years ago, when F— called me up from a camping trip to see whether Arin had been born yet. He had, and F—had news for me; her period was late one day, and she *always* gets them 28¼ days apart. At the time her younger son was 8 months old. Ya hafta know F—. I laughed and said I also thought she was probably preg. And a few weeks later I got a postcard. The message consisted of one word—"preg". Anyway, that's how "preg" got started. Also, when we were kids, R— and I used to say "pred" as short for "pred-judiced." I don't know; it just sort-of developed.)

Anyway, my mind leaps ahead. I so want to be happy again. I so want to mourn Kerin, and not me. I so want to love Kerin more than mourn her.

However, not only does it have to *happen*, but it has to *have* happened! That's even harder. In fact, that's impossible, since it's too late to do anything about it now.

However, if *it* has to happen, or have happened, so did the meconium staining. And *that* happened. So this will, too.

June 15, 1978

It's the night before two weeks after the earliest day I could have ov'd; *i.e.*, it's the night before the earliest day I could get my period (unless I get it early, which I often do). So what I'm doing is enjoying these last few moments of (relative) happiness.

Actually, I'm partially home-free. My waking temp was 98.6^+ this morning, after five hours of sleep (98.4 after seven hours), so it's not very likely I'm gonna get my period tomorrow. In fact, it's also not very likely that it's gonna drop enough for it to be indicative of getting my period the *next* day, either. So that leaves the day after that, or June 4 as ov day, which also isn't very likely. In other words, I could be preg.

June 16, 1978

Okay—here's the scoop.

Last night I awoke, as usual, around 4:00, and slept only intermittently thereafter. I don't know if it's nervousness or

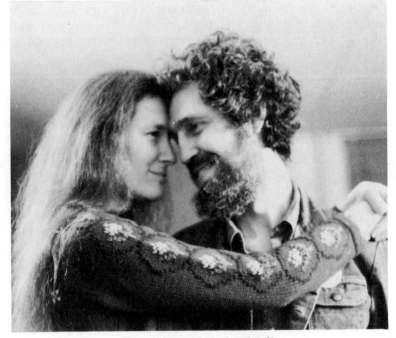

The Author and Husband Jeff

the fact that I went to bed at 11:00 and thus already had five hours of uninterrupted sleep and wasn't particularly tired. Anyway, when I first got up, I didn't feel pre-menstrual at all, but then I started thinking about it and my back started to ache and I felt all loos-ish and my legs even felt crampy. It didn't feel like nerves, but what else could it have beed? I was sure, absolutely sure, I wasn't preg. And I felt miserable. At one point I felt myself sit upright for a few seconds and I felt my period ooze out. "Damn it," I whispered. A second later I rubbed my eyes in surprise. I was lying down and there was no period. I had dozed off and it had been a dream. So I decided to Be Brave and sit upright. And no, there was no period. And, for a second, there were no cramps until I started thinking about it. But it was by now almost 5:00 and I had had almost six hours of sleep/rest. So it was legitimate to take my temp.

Guess what it was?! It was—98.6$^+$.

Yup, 98.6$^+$. Not *as* + as yesterday, but how pretty can you get?! And besides, *this* 98.6$^+$ was after six hours whereas yesterday's 98.6$^+$ was after five hours. So today's is more valid.

So that steps up by one day everything that was true last night, so chances are I won't get my period at all. In other words, chances are I'm preg.

Yes, I admit it—at the risk of God punishing me—I do think I'm preg. (God would punish me anyway.)

Chances are I'm preg, and so I fear the switcheroo. A sudden drop in estrogen, a later period, or a period without a temp drop. No explanation required. No explanation given. God can do whatever he wants. I fear the switcheroo.

Still, chances are that I'm preg. They really are. And I'm so excited, so nervous, and—I admit it—sooo happy. At the risk of God's punishing me, I'm happy.

Oh, I'm still sad about Kerin. But I'm also happy about L'il Fetus. I'm sad *and* happy. It doesn't average out. I'm not half-happy, or half-sad, or both. The happiness and sadness exist side by side, not unconnected, but side by side nonetheless.

Oh, I'm so close. So close to the end of the nightmare. So close. Oh God, so close. No switcheroo, please. Please-oh-please no switcheroo.

I know God won't care if my writing this beats him to the

punch and I know nothing I write here can possibly have an effect upon what happens this weekend. But I *feel* as though it can. I feel as though if only I write the right thing, God will reward me. Or rather, not punish me.

I swear, I'll forget them until I go through them again. The ol' trying-to-conceive days. First I walk around listening for the Spinnbarkeit, feeling for that sponginess every time I go to the bathroom. Then I walk around with semen in my underwear, reminding myself that it's neither Spinnbarkeit nor a period. Then I walk around listening for pre-menstrual cramps, and with sweat in my underwear, continually reminding myself that it's not a period. I swear, I always forget these days.

June 17, 1978

98.6⁻ after eight hours. But I feel crampy again, and Cerv is softening and opening up, possibly to make room for a period.

I'm a nervous wreck. Am I not preg or am I preg and it's just not holding or am I just plain preg? I'd hate to have been preg and not known it. I'd hate to lose a child I never knew about.

Does God have a plan—like in that story by Poe? The guy *thinks* he's escaped the horrible Inquisition death; but then at the last minute he gets captured again. Turns out the whole thing was planned, by the Inquisition, so the guy, having *al*most escaped, is even *more* terrified. Is that what God has planned?

June 18, 1978

Someday. Someday, the nightmare will be over. I just don't know when.

Tonight was virtually sleepless. I was more excited than nervous. I simply couldn't wait to see the high temp the next morning. I just couldn't wait. I didn't even get any cramps because I just wasn't nervous. Aw c'mon, I told myself, you know darn well you're preg. Tomorrow will just complete the weekend. Tomorrow will just be the clincher.

At 2:20, two and a half hours after falling asleep, I awoke and took my temp, just for the hell of it, and found—97.6. But I wasn't too worried, because my temps are usually lowest a short time after I fall asleep. Just for good measure, though, I took my temp at 3:00. It was just under 98. That satisfied me. But, as I said, I couldn't go back to sleep because I was just too excited about L'il Fetus. So I lay there quietly and waited for 5:00! (Don't tell me not to care so much. I already do. And remember—it's easy to be calm when you don't care. That's why children aren't calm.) Well, at 5:00 my temp was 98.2. Not 98.6$^+$, just 98.2. Not super-high, but probably high enough. High enough to see me through the weekend. And besides, it had been slightly chilly in the room. And besides, an hour later my temp was 98.4. Happy and exhausted, I finally fell asleep.

An hour and 45 minutes later I awoke—to 98$^+$. Just plain 98$^+$—borderline. I could get my period tomorrow, or even today.

It's unnerving, that's all. Probably everything's fine. If I weren't preg, I'd've gotten my period by now. I mean, I usually get it less than 14 days after ov-ing. Probably everything's fine. Probably L'il Fetus is in there, and intact. Probably my temp just dropped because of the short deep sleep. Or for some other reason. And remember when I was preg with Elle and it was 97.8. And with Kerin, 97.9? Probably everything's fine. I still *feel* preg. No cramps and Cerv sort-of soft but closed. And remember the 98.4? Yes, probably everything's fine. It's just unnerving, that's all.

Oh, yes, and the reason I took my temp so many times is that I expected another 98.6$^+$ and that would have been reassuring. But now, I don't know. I'll probably be nervous all day. Not to mention tomorrow morning when I take my temp.

Oh, probably everything's fine. It's just that I'm temporarily fearful. It's quite simple, really. Every woman who loses a baby is temporarily fearful. But *really*, there *is* nothing to be fearful *about*. Right? God isn't lying in wait for me. That 98$^+$ was just a fluke. I was especially tired or something. It's just a fluke and it's the 98.4 that counts. In a few days I'll laugh about all this. Everything really is fine. Right? In a few days the nightmare will be over—right?

I think of a poem of mine, a "tidbit":

> *The child said*
> *'I don't wanna wait 'til tomorrow*
> *Or some other time*
> *Because tomorrow means maybe*
> *And some other time means maybe not.'*

Why do I keep looking for things to worry about? Am I a masochist?

No, it's just that I don't want to let God catch me unawares. If he pulls a switcheroo, I'd like it to be *less* of a switcheroo.

June 19, 1978

I *am* preg, right? It's not just a delayed period. There won't be a switcheroo, will there?

This morning, after 5 hours of sleep, my temp was 98.2^+— which is fine. So now I'm still in bed, writing. The fan is blowing on me, but I'm not cold. If anything, I'm a little warm. I'm indulging in some activity, and some more time has past. So you'd expect the temp to go up. But it didn't. In fact, it's only 97.8.

Huh? I asked. It's unnerving. God *couldn't* have planned a switcheroo to end all switcheroos. Could he? It's unnerving. I mean, suppose I hadn't taken my temp before? Suppose I'd taken it only now? Well, then I'd be all miserable.

What's going on? Why did I hafta open up my big mouth and stick in that thermometer?! Why can't I leave well enough alone? Why am I a mathematician? Why am I the "Master of the Long Proof"? That's what they used to call me, in high school. The Master of the Long Proof.

June 20, 1978

Someday, someday, the nightmare will be over. Someday, someday, I know not when.

Apparently not this month. No, *I* didn't believe it, either, but it happened. The switcheroo. It really did happen.

I wish I was masochistic.

Jeff says next time. He says he didn't want it this time, anyway, says he wants a spring baby 'cause spring babies have a better chance.

I say why should it be next time? It wasn't this time and it wasn't the last time. Why next time? Also, next time is a month away.

Someday, someday, the nightmare will be over. I just don't believe it.

I'm not gonna write so much any more. Just in case, subconsciously, I *am* making the switcheroos happen in order to write about them. Or just in case *God's* making them happen so I can write about them. No more writings for you, God. Not until you let me get preg.

I'm a loser, all right. Just not a *good* loser.

June 29, 1978

My state of mind has changed. And it's not good. I mean, it's the end of June. It's been six months. Spring has come and gone, and now it's summer. Jeff's mother's surprise 60th birthday party, my Walt Whitman Center poetry reading, Arin's fifth birthday—all have come and gone. Spring has failed me. Summer has failed me. All of nature has failed me. I can't go on much longer. The nightmare must end. It *must* end. So I have given God an ultimatum: If he tortures me again, there won't be any me around to torture. Oh, I'll be around. I just won't be the same. Some of my mind will be gone. I can't take any more. Oh, I realize it's been *nine* months for Holly of UNITE, but, for me, six months was the limit. I'm *not* a strong woman. My mind is going. I now plead with God *aloud*. "You *must* let it end." "It *must* end. You must give me another chance. I must have the chance."

True, I do a lot of this purposely—an ultimatum, as I said. Also catharsis. But still, that last month took a large chunk out of me. And I can't take any more. If July lets me down, I won't be me anymore. I won't be around for God to torture.

Allison from UNITE called the other night, and we talked for about an hour. And I found out that I'm not unique with this God business. She feels the same way. That makes me feel a lot better, of course, but it doesn't prove that it's all our imaginations. I mean, God could still *really* be purposely trying to torture us.

Some more low-down: Eileen of UNITE had a 7 lb. 7 oz. boy last night. I'm genuinely happy for her. But Lorena, who's one-month old was killed by a dog in January, is almost certain she's preg again. *Her* I feel increasingly jealous of. I mean, *her* baby died *after* mine. BUT: My temp was 97.4 this morning.

June 29, 1978

People who read my *Hera*-article are non-commital. They make no comment at all. I know I'm not imagining it. It happened at the UNITE meeting, and with one of Jeff's friends. They just read it and then talk about something else. Ignore it, in other words.

I betcha people think I'm just a sore loser. They think I'm just mad so I have to blame somebody. Like when I was having trouble getting that PhD. It really *was* Wesleyan's fault, but I betcha they all thought I was just being a bad sport. So now they think I'm just blaming B— because I have to blame somebody. Maybe they even believe B—. Maybe they believe I killed my baby. Maybe I don't fit in even with UNITE.

Maybe they think it's a case of "The lady doth protest too much." But if I *don't* protest, how can they know? Maybe I'm supposed to protest a certain *optimum* amount. How can I know what that amount is?

To everybody I say: B— *did* kill my baby. If B— killed *your* baby, what would you do?

But I don't care if I don't fit in. I don't care about that. I just want God to let me have another baby. As long as I can have a baby. I just want a baby. I just want my baby.

July 1, 1978

I long—how I long—for an end to the nightmare. I long—
how I long—for an end to the ordeal. I long—how I long—for
my life.

Barbara's preg; how I long to be preg *with* her. She *wants*
me to be preg with her. Says she needs somebody to be preg
with, 'cause she's scared, Afraid the baby won't be as good as
her first. *I'm* not scared; I just want a baby; I just want my
baby. The less it sleeps, the better! Oh, how I long for life
again! To laugh, knowing the main thing in my life is okay. To
stop feeling sorry for myself, to stop feeling others feeling sorry
for me. How I long for life—for *my* life. To walk into Dr. Mc's
office as a pre-natal patient. To fill up my maternity smocks,
to eat spinach, to look radiant. How surprised Dr. Mc's will be.
He warns me I can't be expected to enjoy my next pregnancy.
How surprised he'll be, how he'll admire me! How I long for
my vanity—how I long for my life. Until I get baby, baby, I
could settle for my life. I have ideas for baby blankets. A
Kewpie-doll quilt, akin to the Sunbonnet baby quilts. Then,
what I call a 'Fetus-quilt". Each square'll show a different
stage of L'il Fetus' development. In the first, a little cartoon
sperm racing toward a cartoon egg—the sperm in pink if a girl,
blue if a boy. Then a four-week fetus, then a three-month
fetus, then a squawling birthling, then a neonate—complete with
umbilical stub, tied with pink ribbon if a girl, blue if a boy.
"She can look at it that way even though she lost a baby?"
they ll all say. How neat I'll be, how happy I'll be. How I long
for my self, how I long for my life. And a "Fetus T-shirt."
"Baby" it'll say, with an arrow pointing down—only on the
stomach part'll be a simplified slightly-funny, slightly-serious
very sophisticated drawing of L'il Fetus. And then *The Little
Prince*. Another blanket, or maybe a receiving blanket. "The
Little Prince on Asteroid B-12" or "Where I come from, everything is very small"—the original drawing and quote, in machine
embroidery. Oh, God, I promise all this will be in the back-
ground. I promise what I'll mostly do is lie in the sun and *think*
about L'il Fetus and *be* with L'il Fetus. Oh, God, I promise—if
only. . . .

How I long for my mind, how I long for my life. Not
hunger, but thirst. How I long for my life.

I've tried taking my life back with*out* being preg—but it just doesn't work.

July 16, 1978

If, and only if, and when, I get preg will I relate in detail the grueling events of my last (unsuccessful) cycle. Yes, God, only if you come through will your stubborn child of a writer (or *one* of your writers) continue to work for you. Yes, God, I'm going on strike. (A hunger strike, of sorts). For, although I enjoy being different, a writer, etc., I'd rather have a baby. I just want a baby. I just want my baby.

It reminds me of a poem—not one of mine, this time (See, I'm not self-centered)—but one of the poems in the women's anthology Wemara and I put out. "I will not be," she says. "For them, I will not be." The poem is called "No" and the author is 14 years old.

I will not be for you, God. I will not be. Let me get preg and I will be again—for you or for anyone else who wants me. But until then, I will not be.

If this is the last sentence of this diary, then you'll all know I never got preg. Oh, how I hope God doesn't take a fancy to this ending.

August 24, 1978

Dear Eileen and Irv,

I'm finally getting around to sending this off. I hope it's not too small for Kevin by now.

A few weeks ago, I had a revelation, which I'd like to share with you because it seems pertinent for all of us. Remember how we were talking at the UNITE meetings about "the need to know why"? And you were saying you'd never rest until you found out *why?*

Well, I was wondering, "Will we rest even then?" i.e., if we were ever to find out why, exactly why our babies died, exactly why it happened to us, would we be satisfied?

The answer's "no", right? I mean, suppose God (or whoever's in charge) were to actually confront us and give us a per-

fectly logical reason. Would we accept it? Of course not!

But wait; there's more! Then I was thinking about kids, when they asked why. Why can't I have ice cream? Why can't Amy sleep over? Why did you hit me? And if you tell them why, they just repeat "But why?"

No matter how logical the reason, no matter how well you explain it, they're not satisfied. Even if they understand, they aren't satisfied.

Because they don't really want to know why. What they want is for things to be changed. They want to be told, "Well, okay, you can have ice cream. Amy can sleep over. I won't hit you again (no matter what you do)." It's not curiosity on their part; it's a demand for change.

And so with us. Why did it happen? we ask God. If our babies had lived, we wouldn't give a damn why. Why? we ask. But we don't want God to tell us. What we want is for God to say, "Well, I guess there's no really good reason for it to have happened, so I guess it didn't happen!" We don't really want to know why; we just want to put God on the spot so he has to give us our babies back.

Just thought I'd share all that with you. Maybe it'll help. Hope I'm not doing the wrong thing.

Wish I could make another long distance 'phone call like the last one, but can't afford it! Hope you'll bring Kevin to one of the meetings sometime.

Love,
Marion

P.S. I'm four days late (i.e. I ov'd 18 days ago.) and my waking temp's still high. I'm on pins and needles, afraid to be happy. The book says 16 high-temp days is a valid pregnancy test, but I don't feel too trusting this time around. Will let you know if.

September 11, 1978

preg. . . .

preg. . . .

Yup! **PREG!**

PREG

Not 17 months preg! Not minus-two months preg! Not 1%, or 25%, or 50%, preg. But *actually* hones'-t'-goodness bona-fide preg!

Five weeks, to be exact.

Oh, my!

Oh, wow!

WOW!! WHEEE!!!

The nightmare *is* over. Or, if something goes wrong, at least I have a nice long *break* from the nightmare!

Oh, wow!

Oh, oh! wow!

I've almost *forgotten* the nightmare. Not Kerin—just the nightmare. I've almost forgotten it!

And I've got back my life. I've already had the fun of telling our parents, telling Carol and Ruth from UNITE, telling some of the dykes—I felt really proud when K— said, 'Ya know, you're the only woman I'm excited about hearing she's pregnant!'—taking the pregnancy test in Mc—'s office, taking the home preg test (the ring oh, that beautiful, beautiful ring! It's still on our dresser. It's supposed to start disappearing after two hours, but it's been almost six days now! Jeff wants to keep it there during the entire pregnancy), checking up on Mc— via the C.E.A. (he comes very highly recommended), telling some of our friends at the park, calling up Wemara at work as soon as I got home from the positive preg test, and, yes, calling up Freda and saying, first thing, "Preg." (Yes, she knew right away, who it was.) I've already had all those funs. *Now* I have, yet to come, the fun of breaking the news at the next UNITE meeting. of making all those baby items I was writing about, of seeing if zinc really does cure morning sickness, and—of course—my first real appointment with my first high-risk doctor.

I worry about that, a little. Suppose God is still laughing? Suppose Dr. Mc— says my uterus isn't growing?

Of course, the positive home-pregnancy test shows that it's a uterine pregnancy. And I feel uterus-enlarging cramps, and I go to the bathroom a lot more often, and I have a hint of morning sickness, and more than a hint of fatigue. But my breasts aren't enlarging, I remember that they were last time by one month.

Yes, I worry. But not a whole lot. Nothing like before. I don't feel as Kafkaesque as before.

I'm still careful. I worry about bleeding. I wonder about every sensation down there. I check when I go to the bathroom, or when I try on clothes in thrift shops.

And God hasn't completely disappeared, as I thought he would. Sometimes I even think, "I have a feeling God has something terrible planned." But then I tell myself these are just feelings. Perfectly natural feelings, under the circumstances. The *feelings* can't harm L'il Fetus, I say. Sure, I'll worry. But L'il Fetus will grow, just the same, and in 35 weeks I'll have my baby, just like the other UNITE women who are preg. I won't be the exception. God didn't put me in UNITE just to save the law of averages.

I'll have a baby. I'll have my baby. L'il Fetus will actually *become* a fetus, and then a baby. Baby, baby. Oh, baby, baby. I just had a baby and I'm going to have a baby.

INDEX

A
abdomen 68
anesthesia 66
anesthesiologist 97

B
baby 1, 3, 4, 6-14, 17, 19, 21
. . . . 21-25, 29, 31-33, 36-39
. . . 41, 44, 47, 49-52, 54-55
. . . 57, 59-61, 66, 67, 70-74
. . . 77-79, 82-83, 88, 95, 98
. . . . . 99-103, 105, 107-117
Bereaved Parent, The 84
Bettleheim 48
Bible 57, 58
birth . . . 2, 4, 5, 10, 15, 18, 27-28
. . . 31, 38, 42, 50-51, 60, 84
. . . . 91, 107
birth control 94
birth trauma 51
bladder 18
blood pressure 41, 82, 88
brain 18
Braxton-Hicks 10, 11, 13, 41
breast feeding 75, 76

C
Carter's (store) 8, 22, 87
Cervix 71, 80, 105-107
cervical mucus 36
Cesarean birth 38, 60
Chanukah 12
colostrium 40
conception . 10, 24, 32, 34, 35-36
. . . . 38, 44, 47, 51, 69, 103
contraction, birth 10, 13, 15
. . 16, 17, 33, 35, 41, 44, 49
. . . . 76, 78, 80, 81
Crib Death 35

D
*Davis, Adelle 15, 16, 48
delivery . . . 2, 6, 9, 15, 17-18, 21
. . . . 24, 25, 37, 61
Demerol 90
demons . . . 23, 28, 30, 33, 45, 53

dreams 2, 23-24, 35, 39, 46
. . . . 75, 76, 87
Drexel University 4, 103
Dyke Tactics *see* lesbian

E
eclampsia 82
egg 80, 92, 103
episiotomy 10

F
Fallopian tubes 93
fantasy 6, 12, 25
Fate 75
fear 20, 24, 34-36, 42, 45, 46
. . . . . . 47, 49, 59, 84, 103
Feminism . . . 7, 27, 38, 46, 57, 94
fertility 74, 93, 107f
fetal distress 41
fetal heart-beat 74
fetus 92

G
Giovanni's Room (gay/feminist
bookstore, Philadelphia) . . . 7
God . . . 1, 3, 5, 6, 14, 21, 23, 25
. . . . 27-29, 31-32, 35-36, 38
. . . 41-43, 45-48, 55, 57, 59
. . . 60-63, 65-66, 69, 72, 74
. . . . . . 75, 77-80, 106, 107
grief 23, 24, 59, 62-63, 85
guilt 8, 21, 47, 61

H
Health-Tex 80
heart 16, 18, 20, 44, 92, 102
heaven 51, 66, 67
hypertension 82, 84

I
incubator 20
Inquisition 105
Intensive Care Unit 20, 52
IUD 93

J
Jefferson Hospital . . 18, 19, 37, 96

K

Kafkaesque feeling. . .51, 91, 114
Kerin . . .19-28, 30, 32-33, 35-42
.44-46, 51-54, 58-59, 65-69
. .71-72, 77-78, 83-84, 86-90
. . . . . .102, 106, 107, 116
kidneys 18, 20

L

labor. .2, 11, 13, 15-16, 24, 27-28
. 36, 41-42, 44-45, 60-62, 66
. . . . .74, 81, 97
Lesbian 2, 7, 74, 83, 113
Lesbian Center 45
Lesbian Custody 64, 81

M

meconium 4, 13, 15, 16, 18
. . . . . 28, 31, 38, 42, 52, 96
menstruation . . 52, 71, 106, 107
midwife. 9, 104
Miro, Juan 8
Mittelschmerz. 68, 80
monitor. 16, 17, 24, 51, 52
. . . . 97, 100
morning sickness 39

N

natural childbirth 58
Nausea 11
Nembuthol. 90
New Age Baby Book 31
*Nin, Anais 79
nirvana 67
nursing (breast-feeding) . . 13, 27

O

obstetrics. 52
orgasm 4, 80
orgy 23
ovaries. 69, 71, 83
ov *see* ovulation
ovulation. . 24, 36, 51, 57, 62, 65
.67-69, 70, 72, 81, 82, 85-86
. . 87, 88, 102, 107-108, 109
oxygen 16-18

P

PABA 67

paracervical block 60
past-datism. 37-58
pelvic 9
perineum 4
Pit and the Pendulum. 16
Pitocen 37-38, 51, 97, 100
pituitary gland 67, 69
placenta. . . 29, 37, 51, 61, 76, 82
placenta abrupta 74
Poe, Edgar Allen 105
Politics of Motherhood. . . 2, 7, 8
. . . . .57, 58, 88
post-partum . . .18, 25, 27, 28, 40
. . . . 74, 85
preg *see* pregnancy
pregnancy . .1-3, 7, 13, 24, 27-28
. . 33, 35, 37, 39, 40, 41, 45
. . .50, 54, 55, 57, 58, 61-65
. . . 69, 70-72, 74, 75-78, 84
. . 87-88, 91, 93, 95, 97-101
. . . .103, 104, 105, 106-117
Prince, The Little 110
Providence *see* God
pulse. 18

R

Ram Dass, guru. 67
reality 21, 30, 31, 33, 35, 51
. . . . 78, 79
Retarded Children's
Organization. 89

S

*Sartre, Jean 11
Schmerzen. 68
S.E. Press. 15, 58
Seven Woods Press. 67
Shakespeare, William 8, 51
Solipsist. 11, 28-29
sperm 93, 103, 104, 107
Spinnbarkeit. . . 67-68, 79, 81, 89
. . . . .103, 107
sterility (sexual) 38, 81
stethoscope 16
stillbirth 38, 76

T

Temple University 4, 52
Tes-tape. . . 36, 67, 71, 74, 80-81

Tes-tape (*continued*) 89, 93

U

UNITE 55, 61, 71, 74, 87, 89
. . . . . 103, 111, 112, 114, 115
urine analysis 20
uterus 27, 51, 83

V

vitamins. 9, 10, 12, 16, 27, 39
. . . . 48, 54

W

Walt Whitman Poetry Center .38, 108
Wesleyan University. 112
women . . . 2, 4, 5, 6, 38, 40, 46, 50
. . . . 52, 53, 58, 62, 66, 68, 81
. . . . 81. 87, 91, 93

Denotes contemporary author.

ABOUT THE AUTHOR

Marion Deutsche Cohen was born at Perth Amboy, New Jersey. She received her B.A. in mathematics (*magnum cum laude*) from New York University, and M.A. and Ph.D. in mathematics from Wesleyan University. She has held academic positions at New Jersey Institute of Technology, City College of New York, Community College of Philadelphia, and currently at Drexel University and Temple University. A holder of the Phi Beta Kappa key, she has had numerous awards and grants. She actively participates in support groups for bereaved parents (UNITE, SIDS, etc.), and is a contributing editor of *Mothering* magazine.

A poetry contributor and coordinator for many publications and women's groups, Dr. Cohen has published frequently with various presses. She is the mother of four living children, and is the wife of physicist Jeffrey Cohen of Philadelphia.